The Human Side of Nursing

A Short Story Collection

By

Lois Gerber, RN, BSN, MPH

Copyright Information

The Human Side of Nursing: A Short Story Collection
Second Edition

Lois Gerber, RN, BSN, MPH

ISBN: 978-0692298817

Nursing: A Legacy of Service
Making a Connection
Tattooed Poets and Peanut Butter Sandwiches
(Original title: Tattooed Poets and Peanut Butter)
The Home Visit
Blind Faith
Nursing: It's What I Do
(Original title: The Sacred Path)
Watercolors in the Rain
Things Money Can't Buy
The Crisis
The Other Cheek
The Teacher
Beyond the Facade
Two Nurses: One Old; the Other New
Smoked Tinged Glasses
Nurses Know
What Nursing Taught Us

The following [illegible] have appeared [illegible] versions [illegible] published [illegible]
[illegible]

[illegible] Publications

Dedication

Dedicated to all the nurses
throughout the world
and to the patients for whom they cared.

Acknowledgements

The patients and families who taught
me about the important things in life—health, family, friends, and
meaningful work.

My nursing students who reinforced my love of learning and
commitment to share my knowledge.

My writing group members who shared their wisdom and
knowledge.

My writer friend, Mary Jane Forbes,
who guided me through this book's formatting process.

Other Books by Lois Gerber's in her series,
Nursing in the Neighborhoods

Nurses and Their Patients: Acts of Courage and Conviction
Nurses and Their Patients: Courage and Compassion

Table of Contents

NURSING: A LEGACY OF SERVICE

Nurses are the heart of health care.
Donna Wilk Cardillo

Right before I was born, a psychic read my mom's palm. "She'll be a girl, and she'll be a nurse just like you. You said you've been an R.N. for ten years. Nursing is in your blood; it'll be in hers, too. Just wait and see."

***

I am four years old, looking at Mom bathe my little brother, Tommy, in a dishpan of warm soapy water. I didn't know it at the time but he is dying. I watch her hands gently rinse him with a soft washcloth. I marvel how her long sensitive fingers gently touch his skin and how her rubbing his head and back soothes his crying. I observe her squeeze red liquid medicine into his mouth from an eyedropper and then carefully peel tape from his bandage; she pulls so slowly, he doesn't even flinch. I brush my hand across her arm. She looks at me and smiles.

***

I am six years old. "Where did you get this bowl with all the blue and yellow flowers painted on it, Mommy?"

"It's from Johnny Ackley's mother. I took care of him in the hospital before you were born. He didn't have a daddy. His mom worked lots of hours as a waitress. He was only ten. His cousin accidentally shot him in the leg, and the wound got infected. He screamed when I had to stick him with a needle or change his dressing. But afterwards he'd hug me, and I'd make him jelly toast, his favorite snack. His family didn't visit much, but was so excited to take him home. His mom and aunt gave me this bowl because at the time I cared about him more than they were able to."

I pick up the bowl, turn it over in my hands and wonder what Johnny Ackley is doing now. I want to become a nurse when I grow up.

***

I am eleven years old and very shy. Mom is helping Dad, a pharmacist, deliver medications to his clients. "I need you to come with me", she says. "We have to drop off this medicine to people at home too sick to get out. I'll drive, and you'll run the packages up to the doors."

"No," I yell. "I don't want to go to strangers' houses and talk to them. What will I say?"

"Just step inside and smile. Ask them how they are and compliment them on something they're wearing. That's all. Those few minutes you spend talking with them will make them happy for hours."

In the end, I go with Mom, and she is right. Most are ladies, just a few older men, and they smile back and maybe even laugh. Sometimes they pat me on the arm and give me cookies or candy.

***

I am fourteen years old. Grandma has just had a stroke. Her right side is paralyzed, and she can't talk or swallow well.

"Gladys, come over." the aunts say. "We need you."

Mom packs her suitcase and goes. She stays for weeks, coordinating Grandma's care, for the family wanted her to be taken care of at home, not in a nursing home. Mom orders all the equipment - hospital bed, bedside commode, walker, and tub bench. She teaches the aunts and uncles how to care for Grandma, things like arm and leg exercises, getting her out of bed, and feeding her so she didn't choke. Grandma never completely recovers, but she learns to walk and feed herself again.

The aunts are grateful. "We couldn't have done it without you, Gladys."

Mom tells me "Nursing's not just hands on care, it's helping people learn to manage by themselves. When you're a nurse, family and friends look to you for advice. We're good listeners and problem solvers.

***

I am sixteen years old. My early desire to become a nurse has become stronger. At first it was an instinctive feeling, a vague way to connect to others and be like Mom. Now it's a definite career calling.

I accept a summer job as a nurses' aide in the hospital Mom retired from. I'm naïve and innocent when I begin. By the end of the summer, I'm wiser, more street smart. I learn that sick men can act out their sexuality by groping and that their sexual innuendos don't automatically equate with their being perverts. I realize I can control these situations with firm quiet statements like, "Your behavior isn't appropriate. You'll have to stop, or I'll need to call for help."

I learn that life isn't fair; that really nice people get very ill and even die, and that there are no rational explanations. People like Angela Barrio, for instance. She's Italian and recently lost her sight. In between chanting, "Me no can see" in broken English, she asks "Why did this happen to me? Why was I the one who got acid in my face? I must be a bad person for God to treat me this way."

Angela's corneal repair surgery fails. No one knows why her eye rejected the donor graft. She cries almost constantly and refuses to eat. Her face is oily, and her shoulder length hair hangs in greasy strands because she won't wash. She leaves the hospital sobbing, holding tight to her daughter's arm as she staggers down the hall.

***

I am eighteen years old. I'm leaving for college to study nursing. As I'm packing, Mom saunters into my bedroom. "Are you glad you were a nurse?" I ask her.

"Nursing gave me a core to build my life around," she answers. "You know I ran away from home to escape from my abusive alcoholic father. Nursing took me in, accepted me and gave structure to my life. I found strong capable caring friends, all nurses, who became family to me. You remember Dorothy, the army nurse and Stella who worked in the OR. We watched out for each other, vacationed together, played on the same tennis teams. We all had different personalities. Nursing was the glue that held us together. Nursing will enrich your life, too. You'll see. If you're like me, you'll feel like you got much more than you gave."

***

I am twenty-two years old. I just graduated from college with a nursing degree. Community Health is my specialty, not pediatrics like mom. I accept a staff nurse position with a Visiting Nurse Association. I love being out and about, nursing patients on their turf, seeing how they really live and what they do to take care of themselves. Every patient's situation is different. *Am I a community health nurse because Mom made me deliver medicine? Is that where I learned to be comfortable knocking on strangers' doors and entering their homes to provide health care?*

***

I am twenty-nine years old. I reflect on how much wisdom I've gained from my patients. I entered health care as a sheltered young woman, a middle class suburbanite. Nursing expanded my life experiences; taught me to appreciate and honor those different from myself. I witness the dedication and struggles of young single moms, the ambivalences and conflicts of alcoholics in treatment programs, and the vulnerability of the isolated elderly. I notice how different cultures and races have different diets, different ideas on how to discipline children, and different folk beliefs on the best treatments for specific illnesses.

I taste homemade chitterlings, baklava, and borscht soup. learn how to interact with all types of people. When I visit bad neighborhoods, the residents watch out for me from their windows and welcome me into their homes. "Come in. It's so good to have you here." I see patients lying in hospital beds in living rooms; yet, in poor families three or four people may share a double bed. I tramp through dusty hallways piled with clutter. I climb steps in bars to get to apartments on the second floor. When I hear, "The nurse is here." I smile. I'm blessed to be such an important part of so many people's lives.

***

I am thirty-five years old. I've just been injured in a car accident. An ambulance rushes me to the hospital emergency room. My neck hurts.

A nurse keeps an X-ray tech from getting me up from the hospital gurney. "Stop," she says. "If she fractured vertebrae, moving her like that could paralyze her from the shoulders down."

When the X-rays showed that my neck was broken, I gasp. I suddenly realize that I would have been wheel chair bound for the rest of my life if it weren't for this nurse's quick thinking.

***

I am thirty-eight years old. Certain patients stand out in my mind. There's Irma Higgins and her husband, Jim. Both retired early because of Irma's advanced multiple sclerosis. In the beginning, she was very depressed and angry. Now she tutors elementary school children who function below grade level. Irma teaches from a wheelchair in her home using workbooks and personal stories to make her points. She gives the children lots of hugs. Her sessions end with chocolate chip cookies. The kid's schoolwork improves. Irma says finding a way to share her talents, even with illness and disability, has made her life worthwhile. Jim shows me how important committed caregivers are. I realize their task is often harder than the patients.

Mr. Goldman, a tall thin man with a long-lined face and a gray mustache, was a Holocaust survivor. He keeps a kosher kitchen where dairy and meat are kept separate. His recent stroke challenges his mobility. Every day I watch him struggle to perform his physical therapy exercises. Each little improvement gives him hope. In two months he's walking with a cane.

I'm curious about his boyhood in Poland. I ask him about the camps. Tears come to his eyes. "I can't talk about it. My whole family died. Only my sister and I are left. I'd like to tell you, but I can't." Some pain is so deep that there are no words to describe it.

When I visit Mr. Goldman for the last time, he gives me a water-colored still life he has painted of Albert Einstein. Under the sketch, in a shaky hand, he has written, "Without a sense of wonder, life is empty."

***

I am forty-two years old. The white walls of the ICU stare me in the face. Mom is lying unconscious on one of the corner beds hooked up to monitors and IVs. All night long, I have sat bent over by her side, my face buried in a pillow next to her shoulder.

The sheets are wet with my tears. Long forgotten words of Mom's echo in my ears. "Everyone dies when it's the right time. There's a master plan for us all."

Suddenly, her monitor flashes. Her heart has stopped beating. Kathy, her nurse rushes to her side; Dr. Calloway pronounces her dead. I am sobbing. Kathy is holding me and she is crying too. Through her tears, she tells me "Losing a mother is unbelievably painful. It's like losing your life." I cling to her. She whispers, "This is the hard part of nursing made beautiful. Her willingness to face death head-on is an example to us both"

***

It was Mom who taught me that nurses must honor the sacred bond between patients and themselves. Physically caring for someone's body and hearing their deepest secrets builds trust and brings comfort and healing. The great equalizer, sickness, binds us, one to another.

***

Mom's psychic was right. Nursing was in her blood and it's in mine too. Thank God it's a calling neither of us ignored.

TOMMY, THE ANGELS, AND ME

The butterfly counts not months but moments,
and has time enough.

Rabindranath Tagore

When I turned eight, Mama forgot to make my birthday cake. Grandma had to buy one from the store. When Mama, Daddy, and Grandma sang 'Happy Birthday' to me and I blew out the candles, everyone pretended to be having fun.

See, my little brother, Tommy, was very sick. He couldn't walk or play with me, and Mama and I had to feed him mushy food with a special spoon and give him a bath in bed. He couldn't even sit up to blow out three little candles when it was his birthday last week. I had to do it for him.

When I asked Mama what was wrong with Tommy, she said, "We don't know, Lois. Only the angels understand."

Once I heard Aunt Peggy whisper to Uncle Al, "Tommy will never be right." Well, how could Tommy be wrong? He hardly ever even talked.

I hated Tuesdays, the day Dr. McCready came to examine Tommy. The doctor always wore a black suit and looked mean. I didn't like him. He made my stomach hurt. Daddy usually was in a bad mood the day the doctor visited and yelled at me to stay out of the way and not make any noise, not even talking sounds.

Maybe I made Tommy sick when I pinched his leg last Christmas. Maybe that was why he couldn't walk or play with me. I wished I had another brother or sister to talk to about leg pinching. I was too scared to ask Mama or Daddy.

Once when I heard Dr. McCready's car pull into the driveway, I ran into the woods behind my yard and climbed high up into the long branches of a big weeping willow tree. I hid there for a long time chewing on my little finger. I hoped Mama and Daddy would be worried and come outside to look for me. They didn't though, and I finally went back to the house. Mama was standing by the kitchen sink with her back toward me looking out the window. Even though I slammed the screen door, she didn't hear me come in, so I tiptoed upstairs.

Soon, Dr. McCready started to visit more often, because Tommy got sicker. He got thinner and stopped eating or drinking much, even when Mama tried to give him water through a glass straw, but sometimes, he licked sugar from a spoon. The sparkle in his eyes disappeared. He stayed in bed all the time unless Mama or Daddy carried him around.

In the summer, I stayed outside a lot to keep out of everyone's way. My friends, Nicky and Susan, told me I wasn't fun to play with anymore. Most every afternoon, I hid in my special tree.

One day, a lady in a navy blue suit came to see my brother. Her name was Mrs. Harper. She was a nurse, and she visited every week. She was different from Dr. McCready. She smiled and talked to me and let me be in the room with her when she took care of Tommy. She showed me how to wash his face with a small white washcloth. I loved to rinse out the cloth and feel the water in the pan slosh around.

She carried a big black purse with a lot of stuff in it. At first I didn't like her things, but then she told me what they were. "This is a stethoscope," she said. "Do you want to try it?"

"Yeah, I guess."

She pulled back my hair and put it in my ears. At first it felt funny, but then I got to listen to my heartbeat. I liked to hear the thump, thump, thump in my chest.

Some days Mrs. Harper brought me crayons to draw pictures. I drew a big one of Tommy and a little one of me. She asked, "Why did you make yourself small when you're the big sister?"

"Cause he feels bigger."

She sighed. "Hmm. Sounds like you feel small sometimes."

I looked down to the floor.

She knelt beside me and gently lifted my chin so that we were at eye level. "You're very important. Mommy, Daddy, and Tommy need you a lot. You help them smile, just by being you."

I thought about this. "Maybe." I picked up my ball on the floor and bounced it.

Mrs. Harper patted my head. "They're lucky they have you around."

***

One morning when I got up, Tommy wasn't in his bedroom. I hunted for Mama and found her in the living room. "Where's Tommy?" I asked.

"Sit down, Lois," she said. I could feel my heart beating fast.

Mama looked me right in the eyes and whispered, "Tommy's with the angels now. He's very happy. We won't see him for a long time." She stopped talking for a few minutes.

I figured she wanted me to say something, but I didn't know what. I looked down at my feet.

"Why would he go away?"

She said, "It's for the best. The angels wanted him."

"Why can't I have him?"

"The doctor couldn't make him better."

"How come?"

"Sometimes questions don't have answers. I wish they did. I have to go out with Daddy now. Grandma's in the kitchen, and she'll stay with you."

Mama wouldn't look at me anymore, and I knew she wouldn't say anything else and that I shouldn't ask any more questions. She glanced out the window, grabbed her gray purse off the coffee table, and walked out the door to get in the car with Daddy.

I ran back to the bedroom to make sure Tommy wasn't hiding under the blankets. I couldn't find him anywhere. I rushed out to the front porch and sat on the top step and waited for him to come home. For the whole rest of the summer, I sat on the same step every day after lunch and watched for Tommy to walk up the street. I thought maybe the angel would come with him and tell me why he was sick for so long and why he went away.

***

One afternoon in September, when I was sitting on the steps, Aunt Peggy drove up the driveway. When she got out of the car, I noticed her crooked smile right away.

Hugging me, she said, "Hi, Lois. You look pretty today. Maybe the two of us can talk after I see your mom."

"Okay." I opened the door for her to go inside.

When she came out, I was still there. "Lois, what are you doing still sitting on the steps? Are you waiting for someone?"

"I'm waiting for Tommy," I replied. "Mama said he went to heaven with the angels but that we'll see him someday."

She sat down beside me. "Oh, Lois. I can see you're sad. You miss your brother, and that's okay. Tommy can't come back to see you."

"How come?"

"His body won't let him."

I started to cry. "Why?"

"He died. His body stopped working, just like those brown leaves that fall from your special tree."

"But where is he now?"

"Now he lives is in your heart."

I tapped my chest. "How can he be in here?"

"Because you can remember him anytime you want. When you think of him, you'll see his face in your head."

I tested her idea. I thought of him, and he appeared in my mind. He was smiling, and his eyes were sparkly. "I can see him!" I told her.

"You can always see him that way. But you can't see him with your eyes anymore like you could when he was alive, but he'll always be with you."

"I get scared, Aunt Peggy. Mama and Daddy get upset when I ask questions about Tommy."

"Mama and Daddy don't answer your questions because they are so sad they can't talk about him. They miss him too."

"They're mad at me. They think I made him get sick."

Aunt Peggy hugged me tight, and when she pulled back, I saw a tear in the corner of her eye. "No, Honey, you didn't do anything to make Tommy sick. No one knows why Tommy had a bad growth in his brain. It made his body slowly stop working, and then he died."

"No, I did it. I made him sick. When I pinched him, he cried, and Daddy said I hurt him. He yelled at me."

I stood up and kicked the back of the steps. I rubbed my eyes, and Aunt Peggy handed me a tissue. I bunched it up and threw it on the ground.

"Lots of kids get pinched, you know. They don't get sick."

"No, he got sick right after that."

Aunt Peggy put her hands on my cheeks and turned my face toward her. She looked at me with her dark brown eyes. "I promise you, Lois, the pinching had nothing to do with Tommy getting sick."

"I wish I didn't pinch him."

"Lots of big sisters pinch little brothers sometimes. Tommy forgot about it quickly. He knew you were sorry."

"I shouldn't have pinched him though. Daddy said he was special. Why was Tommy the special one and not me?"

"Daddy and Mama think you're very special."

"Then, why did Tommy get to eat sugar right from the spoon and sleep in Mama and Daddy's room at night?"

"Mama and Daddy knew his head hurt, and they wanted to make him feel better. They would have done the same for you if you were sick."

"Why did he go away, somewhere he can never come back from?"

"I don't know, sweetheart. Maybe his life here was finished. The part of him that you remember will always live. The important person now is you."

"No, nobody likes me anymore."

"We'll talk more about how you can be happier. Next time I visit, I'll bring you a present."

"What will you bring?" I smiled.

"Maybe some tulip bulbs to plant in the woods by your special tree. When we first put the bulbs in the dirt, you won't see anything growing. Next spring though, green leaves will peek through the ground and after that, beautiful flowers."

"What color will they be?"

"All different colors. Just like both you and Tommy have many different parts to who you are. Think of Tommy as a tulip – a beautiful brother not with you very long. When he died, he started to live in a new way, a way that's hard for you to understand. Life can be hidden. The tulip bulbs are alive under the ground even though you can't see them now. Tommy's alive now in a way that you can't see."

"Will I get sick like Tommy?"

"You're strong and healthy and very special. Your body's not like Tommy's"

"Will I die, too?"

"Someday we will all die like Tommy, and people will miss us too like you miss Tommy. I think your body will live for a long time."

***

When I turned nine, Tommy wasn't there to watch me blow out my candles. Now I understood that Tommy would never come back to play with me, and I stopped sitting on the steps. Months later the tulips that Aunt Peggy and I planted sprouted. One April afternoon, I saw three green leaves. Soon there were bright red, pink, and yellow flowers. I watered them almost every day until the petals died and fell off the plant. I called them "Tommy's Tulips." That's when I started to play with my friends, Nicky and Susan, again.

For a while I thought the angels had forgotten me. I never saw anyone floating around with white robes or heard voices from the sky. But maybe some angels live on earth and are aunts or nurses, wear regular clothes, and talk like normal people. Maybe Mrs. Harper and Aunt Peggy were two of those kinds of angels.

When I get big, maybe I can be an angel, too. Or maybe a nurse like Mrs. Harper.

MAKING THE CONNECTION

To win without risks is to triumph without glory.
Cornielle

Crashing a World Series game taught me a different way to communicate with patients.

In October, 1960, I was a nursing student at the University of Pittsburgh. The New York Yankees were in town to play the Pittsburgh Pirates. At the end of our clinical day, two friends and I decided to crash the Series seventh game. We rushed back to the dorm to return our nursing caps and aprons. Still wearing our navy blue student uniforms, we ran the half-mile to Forbes Field, the ballpark, pushed through the stile and inched our way to the box seat section. Already the middle of the eighth inning, the Pirates were two runs behind.

By the bottom of the ninth, the Pirates were at bat with two men on base when Bill Mazeroski hit a home run to give Pittsburgh a ten-nine victory. We joined the throngs of people rushing onto the field—newspaper reporters, the players themselves, and photographers—shouting, screaming, and waving banners.

The next morning I was back in the hospital at seven. As I rushed past my nursing instructor's office, she called, "Lois, please come in."

Miss Gleason, sitting erect in her starched uniform, removed her horn-rimmed glasses and laid them on her desk next to a newspaper opened to the sports page. Clearing her throat, she stabbed her finger at a photo of my friends and me on Forbes Field, wearing baseball hats and waving our arms.

I wanted to cover my face with my hands. Instead I looked up and forced my eyes to meet hers.

Her voice was firm. "You want to be a nurse, a professional, and this is how you act? You've embarrassed me and the university. Wearing Pitt's nursing uniform to a baseball game and jumping up and down on the field like a crazy person. I never expected you to behave this way."

"I'm sorry. It won't happen again."

"Of course it won't happen again. Another world series in Pittsburgh. Not a chance."

A twinkle shone from her blue eyes, but her face remained stern.

"Can you take over Eddie Hatchett's case?" she asked. "He'll be a good patient for you. He's angry and depressed. Doesn't talk much, only nods and shrugs with lots of yes and no answers."

"Sure," I lied. "I'd like that." Eddie had gone through three nurses already—a strikeout—and I didn't want to be the next one. But to appease Miss Gleason, I wanted to act enthusiastic.

She stood up. "That's all, Lois."

Twenty-six year old Eddie Hatchett—fractured femur, cracked pelvis, bedridden in a partial body cast from a motorcycle accident. He'd be on bed rest for four more weeks. Typically I could get shy patients to talk but not angry, sullen ones like Eddie.

All this was on my mind when I entered Eddie's room to find a thin but muscular man with hazel eyes. His white plaster cast began in the middle of his chest and covered his right leg and the upper part of his left one. As I introduced myself, a faint smile lit his pale face.

He pointed to the newspaper on his bedside stand. "So you're the one. The nurses are talking about you. Looks like you were having fun."

I nodded. My instructor's words about therapeutic communication echoed through my head like the crowds cheering at yesterday's game. *Focus on the patient, not yourself. Direct the conversation toward client-oriented goals. Avoid every day chit-chat. Ask questions—open ended ones to enhance the relationship.*

Smiling, I asked Eddie, "How do you feel?"

"Bad."

"What's wrong?"

"Everything."

"Like what?"

He looked away.

More and more uncomfortable with his short monosyllabic answers, I stopped asking questions and focused on my nursing tasks—checking the skin around the cast edges for redness and infection, taking his vital signs, and turning him on his side to change his bed sheets. "The skin around your cast is clean, no irritation. The blood pressure's fine—118/68. Your foot pulses are strong."

Finally, he looked at me. "Say something useful."

I felt my face flush. Should I disregard my nursing instructor's rules and talk about myself to gain his trust? Or should I ask him more open-ended questions? After glancing at the newspaper on his stand, I decided to tell him about my day at the World Series— the way Mazeroski's ball soared over the left field wall, the runners rounding the bases, and the excitement we spectators felt breaking down the guardrails and stomping out onto the field. I described the trolley ride down Fifth Avenue through streams of confetti, the street and restaurant party celebrations, and sneaking back into the dorm because we'd missed our curfew.

His eyes brightened, and a smile crossed his face. "Wish I could've been there."

I took a deep breath, relieved he was responding. "A once-in-a-lifetime thing. It could happen to you, too."

"I played high-school baseball. Was voted most valuable player my senior year."

"You must have been good," I said.

"Not really, but I love the game. I want to get back on the sandlot team with the guys at work."

"Where do you work?"

"The J &L steel mill, tending the open-hearths. It's darn hard— the blazing hot ovens and heavy lifting. Boring, too."

"Thinking about going back?"

He shrugged.

As the days passed and I followed Miss Gleason's rules about therapeutic communication, Eddie answered most of my questions. I listened intently; encouraged he was talking, even if his voice sounded flat.

"I know it's nuts," he said one day "but I'm scared I'll fall out of bed when the nurses turn me even with the side rails up."

"Trusting someone else to do basic things for you is tough, something you're not used to."

"Everything about this is something I'm not used to."

Miss Gleason met me in the hall that day. "Keep up the good work with Eddie."

"Thanks," I said, hoping she'd forgotten the baseball incident.

As the week went on, Eddie talked more and more openly. Our words became the baseball thrown between a pitcher and catcher practicing for a big game.

He shuddered describing how his motorcycle hydroplaned on wet pavement into a semi. "All of a sudden I was lying on the side of the road, thought I was dreaming. Then I hear these sirens and this EMT guy is staring at me with a terrified look. That's when I realized I was hurt bad. I'll never forget his face. They brought me here in an ambulance."

One day his respiration rate was nearly forty, two times what it should have been. "I feel trapped in this cast like I'm going to suffocate."

After I taught him deep breathing and relaxation exercises and how to lift himself and shift positions using his overhead trapeze, he calmed down.

When I entered his room another day, tears filled his eyes. Squeezing his hand, I asked, "What's going on?"

"My boss was in to visit. He's not sure how long he can hold my job open. Scared the bejesus out of me. I don't know any other kind of work."

"I'm so sorry."

He ran his hand through his auburn hair. "I was too upset to tell him the doctor said two or three more months."

"There's a lot for you to think about. Tell him another day."

"My baseball buddy visited too. The team's saving my spot at shortstop. I pretended I'd be back in top shape." He looked down and patted his cast. "What if it doesn't heal right? I used to be a good runner. Now maybe I'll be a cripple."

"The doctor's very positive."

Over the next month, I learned even more about Eddie. How he'd just met a new girl he thought he wanted to marry, how his younger brother had cerebral palsy, and how his mother baked the best apple pie in the world.

Eddie healed. I fed him as he lay flat in bed and helped him wash his face and arms from a basin of water. I rubbed his back and reinforced the upper body range of motion exercises the physical therapist had ordered.

There was relief in his voice when he told me his boss had agreed to keep him on, even give him a less strenuous job.

After his cast was removed, he was shocked to see the withered muscles in his leg but then excited when X-rays confirmed the bones had mended properly.

Eddie shook my hand the day he was transferred to the rehabilitation center. "Thanks for everything. You helped me a lot."

I swallowed hard. "It worked out for both of us."

Miss Gleason stood in the corner of the room watching us over her horn-rimmed glasses. She nodded her head.

Therapeutic communication. Sure, there are basic principles. As an experienced nurse, I follow them most of the time. But I've learned that you can't always stick to the rues if you want to communicate effectively with your patients. Sometimes, you have to step out of the box and take an unconventional approach,

Like talking about a World Series game to make a connection with Eddie.

TATTOOED POETS
AND PEANUT BUTTER SANDWICHES

By learning, you will teach; by teaching, you will understand.

Latin Proverb

The orientation was finally over. Now my new job as a public health nurse would officially start. I sat with the five other orientees listening to morning report and our instructions for the day.

"Don't forget the brown bag lunch at noon in the conference room," the health center manager reminded us. "You'll meet the Board of Directors there." I fidgeted in my chair anxious for the meeting to end, wondering if I would enjoy working in this busy inner city health department. I was apprehensive about the luncheon too, more boring small talk and worry about appearing friendly yet professional.

Last night, after I made the kids peanut butter and jelly sandwiches, I prepared a tuna pasta salad with croissant rolls to take to the "Get acquainted" meal. I knew a good impression would be important.

"You'll be assigned a supervisor in a few minutes," the manager announced. My ears perked up, wondering which one of the three supervisors I'd be placed with. All six of us orientees had been observing them for the last month.

First there was Mrs. Pitts. We all wanted to be on her team. She had a trim figure and wore her long red hair pulled up into a fashionable bun. Her quick wit and entertaining communication style appealed to us. It was rumored she had a lackadaisical work attitude, but we didn't worry about that.

Our second choice was Miss Perkins, a middle aged spinster, chubby with a Pillsbury doughboy face and short flyaway blonde hair. Because she was kind and non-demanding, we overlooked her disorganization. She flitted from task to task, accomplishing things in a slow roundabout way.

Last, came Mrs. Monroe. Tall with erect posture, short cropped salt-and-pepper gray hair emphasized her organized approach to nursing care. Her crisp navy blue uniform and sturdy black tie-shoes seemed unfashionable and out-of-date for a woman in her forties. Her co-workers respected her competence, but we were scared of her clipped and direct retorts. Staff called her a 'relentless taskmaster' behind her back.

I groaned inwardly when the manager announced that I was assigned to Mrs. Monroe's team.

When Mrs. Monroe called me into her office several minutes later, my heart beat like a jackhammer. "Sit down," she said, looking me in the eye. "Welcome to the team."

"Thanks, I'm glad to be here," I murmured.

"By now you've learned that nurses treat the family as well as the patients. Often, new nurses focus on the social interaction more than the family's health needs. We are not here to be friends to our clients; community health nursing is a professional role. From watching you during orientation, I sense that you agree."

"I do agree," I stammered.

Mrs. Monroe glanced at the calendar on her desk. "I'm going to make shared home visits with you today. We have three clients to see. Here are the charts. Review them and write out for me what you plan to do. Don't forget to check the map. We don't want to get lost."

"Okay. When do you want to leave?"

"Forty-five minutes."

I reviewed the charts quickly. Fortunately, I had my care plan outline completed and the directions to each home plotted out by the time Mrs. Monroe approached my desk. I grabbed my nursing bag, stocked with soap, paper towels, a stethoscope, and other supplies.

"Can you drive?" she asked.

I took a deep breath before agreeing, embarrassed that my small Ford was dusty, and my kids' toys were scattered across the back seat. Mrs. Monroe didn't seem to notice. I hoped she didn't see my trembling leg as my foot released the clutch to shift gears. When I asked for directions to the patient's home, she pointed to the city map on my dashboard. My stomach churned.

First we visited Mr. Franklin, a forty-eight year old single gentleman who lived with his sister in a small two-bedroom upper flat. He needed an intra-muscular penicillin injection for primary syphilis. After I introduced myself, washed my hands, and took his vital signs, I started to draw up the medication in the syringe. My hands began to shake. I turned my back hoping Mrs. Monroe wouldn't notice.

She cleared her throat. "Talk with Mr. Franklin. Tell him what you're doing and why. You're doing fine. I'll sit here out of the way. If you need anything, ask."

Mr. Franklin nodded with an understanding look in his eyes. "You're new. It's okay." He pulled a loose- leaf notebook from his shirt pocket. With a stubby pencil, he started to write, "I write poems for fun," he said. A few minutes later, he handed me the sheet of paper. I looked down and read:

The nurses often come to me with needles long and thin,
And flip me on my stomach so they can stick my lower end.
They rub a spot so very hard, I think that I'll be lame.
But that's the spot so good and red that they must use for aim.
So, if you see me standing, don't think that I'm a boor,
Just think of me as the man the nurses keep so sore.

I laughed, and the hand trembling stopped. After I gave Mr. Franklin his injection, we talked. "I got the sores from that old ho down the street. But, to be honest, I probably spread it to another lady. She doesn't know."

"Really, what's her name?" I asked in a soft voice.

"Jean Krampert. I didn't tell the clinic worker, but I'm tellin' you. I like you." He gave me Jean's address and phone number. "You call her and tell her what she needs to do. I can't. I don't want to see her no more."

"Thanks. We'll check everyone you've had sex with," I said. "Syphilis spreads easily."

"There ain't no one else," he said. "Two women are two too many."

I described how serious syphilis could be, that it could cause blindness, heart disease, and even death unless it was treated with an antibiotic. At times my voice quavered. I waited for Mrs. Monroe to correct something I had said or expand on my ideas, but she never did.

He listened intently and then asked, "While you're here, nurse, my sister's in the other room. Would you look at her finger?"

"Sure, I'd be glad to."

"She has a big pimple where we took out a splinter last week. Does she need an antibiotic too?" He laughed, and then hollered, "Ethel, the nurse is here. She wants to see your finger."

Ethel shuffled into the room and sat down on the sofa. I looked up at Mrs. Monroe, but her head was turned away from me. Realizing I was on my own, I said a bit too loudly, "Let's see what's going on."

The pimple was an abscess, red, swollen, and nearly the size of a quarter. Mrs. Monroe walked over to look at it, and we agreed it needed to be drained.

"Can you call the clinic doctor?" I asked Ethel.

"I guess," she answered. "I won't have to have a shot like him, will I?" she asked with downcast eyes and a trembling upper lip.

"Probably not, pills should clear that up fine," I answered.

"I'll take her. Don't worry," Mr. Franklin said.

As we left the man's apartment, Mrs. Monroe took my arm. "You did very well." she told me. "Besides teaching him about the long term effects of syphilis, you got the name of a contact he wouldn't share yesterday with the clinic nurse. Plus you showed interest in his sister. Like I mentioned earlier, it's important to look at the family, not just the patient."

I smiled and breathed a sigh of relief. "I liked Mr. Franklin, his sister too."

"Good. Let me tell you a story about an abscess. When I worked as a school nurse in a grade school, a boy, about ten-years-old, came in with a huge abscess on his leg. I called his mother and asked her to take him to the clinic. When I saw the child the next day, the abscess had disappeared."

"Wow, his mother listened to you and got him to the doctor fast."

"Not really. When I asked the boy how the doctor's visit went, he told me he didn't see a doctor. He described how his grandmother put warm mashed potatoes on the abscess to draw out all the pus. I was amazed."

"That sounds dangerous," I said.

"It's not a recommended treatment, that's for sure. In his case, the potatoes acted as a poultice. He was lucky. Sometimes, home remedies aren't all bad."

"Sometimes, they make people sicker though," I said.

"Yes, you're right. We have to know what works and what doesn't. Best not to criticize people's folk medicine unless it will hurt them."

"I have a lot to learn."

Mrs. Monroe smiled. "Do you have any questions?"

"I noticed some bugs around the kitchen sink."

"Oh, the roaches. Next time you go, you can talk to the Franklin's about getting rid of them."

"Shouldn't we have said something today?" I asked.

"Best to handle things a bit at a time, unless it's a big concern. The roaches have probably been there for months."

"I've heard about roaches but never have seen them."

"Roaches are a problem in the inner city. We try to get the landlords to treat the whole building, but they balk. And if we report them to environmental health, they evict the families and that can be a worse crisis."

"Nothing's simple, is it?"

"Working with people is seldom simple. We'd better get back for lunch. We'll finish the visits this afternoon."

We drove back to the health center talking more about home remedies. Mrs. Monroe told me how some new moms put one-inch bellybands around their infant's stomachs after the cord comes off. "On the outside of the bellyband, they tape a quarter wanting to keep the belly button from protruding. The quarter's not the problem, but occasionally the skin under the band becomes irritated," Mrs. Monroe said. "Unless there's a bad reaction, we seldom say anything."

Minutes before noon, we pulled into the health center parking lot and got out of the car. I ran to my locker and grabbed my lunch bag. Just in time, I entered the boardroom and set the bag down on the polished oak table. Mrs. Monroe followed behind me with a Tupperware container of chicken Caesar salad. The others had appealing food; I knew my salad would present well, too.

When I opened my bag, I smelled peanut butter! I gingerly pulled the sandwich from the bag and tried to hide it under a napkin.

"Would you like to share my Caesar?" Mrs. Monroe asked.

"Thank you," I responded. "Would you like half of my sandwich?"

"Yes, I love peanut butter and jelly. It's healthy, lots of protein."

When she smiled and winked at me, my hesitancy about working with her dissolved. She might be demanding, but she was kind and insightful and willing to teach me all she knew about community health nursing. I smiled back and joined in the boardroom conversation.

As the day ended, I realized how wrong I'd been about her. My initial perceptions of supervisory figures were often incorrect because of my own fears and insecurities. Mrs. Monroe wasn't a 'relentless taskmaster' but a serious professional nurse who wanted only the best for her patients and the nurses she supervised.

THE HOME VISIT

The doors we open and close each day
decide the lives we live.

Flora Wittemore

On a hot summer day, I sat in my little black Ford looking up at the four-story apartment building. Parked on the side of a quiet street, I was waiting until two o'clock, the time I had scheduled to make my initial visit to Mrs. Lufts, and her new baby, Shannon. I had just started my new job as a public health nurse for the city of Detroit. My mind wandered back to my days as a nursing student.

I thought of my old public health nursing professor, Ms. Powers. I loved the way she talked with patients, and I strove to be just like her. Her easy going, friendly, and upbeat manner acted as a backdrop to her clinical competence. She smiled a lot, called people by name, and asked the right questions to get them talking about themselves before they knew what was happening. Trim and attractive, Ms. Powers always dressed in well-tailored suits and dresses. I never saw her in a nurse's uniform. No matter what the assignment, she wore high heels.

Ms. Powers made shared home visits with all of her students to evaluate our performance. I remembered the day she made a home visit with me. My patients back then were a seventeen-year-old girl, Helena, and her two-month-old baby, Hannah. I had visited them four times by myself and was teaching Helena how to take care of Hannah—the same thing I planned to do with Ms. Lufts and Shannon.

Helena and Hannah lived in a third story apartment above a bar, *The Comfort Café,* loud, noisy, and smoky even in the daytime. To get to Helena's place, I had to walk through the bar and up three flights of rickety wooden steps. I had gotten into the habit of tiptoeing along the café's side wall without saying a word to anyone, so I wouldn't draw attention to myself. I felt more comfortable being on the sidelines.

I wondered what Ms. Powers would think about the rough company and the broken and cracked stairs; she always wore those high skinny heels. What if she tripped? Would she fail me?

I shouldn't have worried. Ms. Powers walked right into the bar and said to the aging bartender with the wrinkled face, "I'm Jennifer Powers, Lois' nursing instructor. I decided to come with her today. I like your neon sign outside. Pink's my favorite color."

She smiled broadly at the younger patrons in their dirty jeans and sweatshirts sitting on the barstools and asked, "Did you see the Steeler's game last week-end?"

An unshaven man with slicked down oily hair and a cigar between his thick lips replied, "I lost fifty goddamn dollars betting on that stupid team." Then, he laughed loudly, cigar ashes cascading to the floor.

Wow, I thought, hurrying after Ms. Powers as she cut a path through the crowd toward the stairway. This is neat.

Ms. Powers took the steps in stride even with her heels. As we started up, I said, "You talked with those men so easily. I wish I could talk to strangers so naturally."

She replied, "Everyone has their own special way with people. You have to find out what yours is; my way may not be your way."

"I like working with people in their homes and seeing how they really live," I said. "Hopefully, I'll learn."

She paused. "Connect with the people you come across in the community in a positive honest way. Meet them where they're at and start conversations about things that interest them."

Then, she gave me some advice I've never forgotten. "Be open to new experiences with the patients and their families, and keep your eye on what's going on around you."

As we reached my patient's doorway, she turned toward me and said kindly, "Don't worry. You'll be a wonderful public health nurse."

Remembering Ms. Powers' words jolted me out of my reverie and back to the present. I took a closer look up and down the Detroit street. In front of an old clapboard two-story duplex, a little boy, dressed in just an old pair of stained green shorts, was kicking a garbage can that lay by the side of the road. A thin expressionless woman with long uncombed hair walked behind him pushing a sleeping toddler in a squeaky stroller.

A construction worker in jeans and a red t-shirt walked out of the building where my new patient lived. He almost crossed paths with an older heavyset balding man in a wrinkled suit just entering the apartment complex.

I looked at my watch. It was almost two o'clock. I picked up my black nursing bag from the passenger seat, stepped out of my car, and walked up the sidewalk. The heavy outer door of the apartment building creaked when I opened it.

The inside hallways were dark. It took a minute for my eyes to adjust to the dim light. When I could see where I was, I started to climb the stairs, three flights of paint worn steps with dust and cobwebs in the corners and around the burned out light bulbs. I arrived on the third floor a little out of breath. I squinted at the doors, but there were no numbers painted on the apartment units. I walked around and listened for noise or people talking. Hearing nothing, I decided to go downstairs. Maybe I had gotten the number mixed up. Maybe it really was 211.

I descended the stairs quickly and went through the door to the second floor hallway. And there it was, Apartment 211. Better yet, I heard people talking behind the closed door. "I was right all along. I had just gotten the number wrong," I whispered to myself.

I knocked loudly on the door. A middle aged blonde woman in a long flowing peach-colored chemise cracked the door open. I peered inside. There sat three gentlemen on soft leather padded chairs. I recognized the heavy middle aged man who had entered the apartment building earlier. He gaped at me from behind his thick glasses. What is going on? In an instant, I knew. Oh, no, a brothel.

Who would have expected to find this kind of business going on the third floor of a dingy apartment in the middle of the afternoon? Was this the type of new experience that Ms. Powers talked about?

Right then and there, I decided, yes, it was and that this would be a day I'd never forget. I smiled at everyone in the room and said, "I'm the baby nurse looking for Mrs. Lutz. Do you know where Apartment 311 is?"

"Yes," the madam said. "It's upstairs right above this unit. There aren't any numbers on the doors up there."

Then, she leaned closer and whispered, "You won't say anything to anybody, will you? You know like the police or anyone."

What would Ms. Powers have done? I remembered another one of her teachings. *Sometimes, it's best to leave things be*, I imagined her saying.

I replied to the madam, "No, I'm just interested in mothers and babies. Thanks for being so helpful. I never would have found the right place without you." She took a deep breath and hugged me.

I walked back up the stairs and suddenly realized the shock I must have had on that small group. And how much I had learned about real life in the short time I had been working. How funny! Still laughing to myself, I knocked on the door to 311.

In the background, I heard a woman's voice say, "Are you the nurse? I'm coming. I'm coming."

BLIND FAITH

Adversity is the diamond dust heaven polishes jewels with.
Robert Leighton

Angela, one of my first home health care clients, taught me that amazing things are possible when nurses, patients, and families work together. To help Angela, I had to walk in her shoes, step to her rhythm, sometimes lead, sometimes follow, and sometimes stumble along beside her. At times it seemed like nothing changed.

Angela, two years away from retirement, was blinded from corneal scarring, the result of a chemical burn at the factory where she worked. Two corneal grafting attempts to restore her vision failed. Her physician wanted her admitted to a nursing home for rehabilitation and then enrolled in a program for the visually impaired. She refused and instead moved into the spare bedroom of her daughter's ranch home.

Several days after Angela's hospital discharge, I met her daughter, Maria, who said, "I need to talk to you before you see Mama."

"All right," I answered.

"I've had it," she lamented. "All Mama says is 'Me no can see'. She's driving me crazy. I want to scream 'shut up,', but I can't. I love Mama too much for that." She pulled a tissue from her jeans pocket.

"Sometimes it's harder to be a caregiver than a patient," I told her.

"If only this accident wouldn't have happened. It's been devastating. My life's been turned upside down."

"It's tiring to take care of a parent." I put my arm across her shoulder. "We'll find ways to make it easier."

"I'm sorry to complain, but Mama was full of life before the accident," she said as she led me into Angela's bedroom. "Her rose garden, the Italian club, she loved it all. Her eyes used to twinkle; now they just stare into space."

I found Angela sitting in her rocking chair. She wore a coffee-stained blue flannel bathrobe. Her downcast dark brown eyes, furrowed brow, unkempt salt and pepper gray hair, and crinkled complexion spoke louder than words. "Robe good enough, more comfortable," she told me. "Me no can see. Me blind now, *cieco.*"

"I know. It was a horrible accident. I'm here for you." I took her hand, and she squeezed my fingers tightly.

On the next visit, I talked privately with Maria and learned how overwhelmed she felt. "Taking care of Mama is too much for me, showering and feeding. I hate eating with her, because food dribbles down her chin when she tries to use a spoon or fork, but she shoves my hand away when I try to help."

"It's good to let her try to do it herself. We can get special silverware for her."

"Those padded handled forks might work with pasta. That's mostly all she wants. Sometimes I cry when I remember how she used to stand over the stove stirring her special spaghetti sauce. She can't do that now."

"You've had a loss, too," I said.

"Loss and stress. Whatever room I go into, she calls out, 'Maria, Maria, me no can see'."

"She's had a terrible shock. She scared, depressed, and you're picking up the pieces."

"Yes, her accident dominates our home. There's no normal conversation anymore."

I obtained physician orders for a home health aide, occupational therapist, and social worker and had the dosage of Angela's anti-depressant medication increased. Within a few weeks, Angela started to brush her teeth, walk from the bedroom to the kitchen, and eat oatmeal with milk and sugar.

One day, Maria told me, "Dr. Guthrie wants to try again, another graft on her right eye. He thinks there's a slim chance for success." She sighed. "Mama won't hear of it."

I asked Angela why she didn't want the surgery.

Her answer surprised me. "No, blindness, my punishment for not being there when Papa die, pass to other side."

"Maria says you took excellent care of her father, I protested."

"I want to hold him when angels come, but I fall sleep in chair. When I wake up, he gone. God's will I must suffer."

Maria stroked her mother's arm. "You did everything for Papa. You bathed him in bed every day and made special soups from the old country recipes. Try the new operation, please," she pleaded.

"Ah, Maria. You ask too much. I ache to see grandbabies faces again, see how grow, but *ospedale* make eyes hurt. Little Frankie, almost four already." She ran her fingers over Maria's face. Tears streamed down her weathered cheeks, as she ran her fingers over Maria's face and through her hair. "I do most anything you want. But no more *ospedale*. Blindness, for me to bear. God's will."

"Just see what the doctor says, Ma. That's all. You don't have to do anything else," Maria begged. "Do it for the grandbabies and me. We love you. We want you to see."

"No, Maria. Leave me alone."

I called Angela's old parish priest, Father Anthony, and asked him to visit. He came the following day. They talked for an hour.

On my next visit, her voice was raspy. "Father Anthony say God want me to see, use doctors for eyes. He and me pray, for first time it feel right."

"You sound sure," I say. "I'm glad."

She nodded. "I feel fear. See, hands shake."

I laced my fingers through hers and hugged her until she stopped trembling.

The surgery was scheduled in five weeks. Angela wrung her hands frequently during the wait. Her shiny black rosary beads seldom left her side. Often times, when she wasn't clicking the beads and saying, "Hail Mary, Mother of God, pray for us sinners," she was chanting, "Me no can see."

A week before the operation, Angela told me, "I dream last night. Angel in white robe come, say, 'Be peaceful, no matter what, I be with you. Remember in heaven you see with soul, not eyes'."

"It sounds like the dream comforted you."

"I different now. Calmer. Worry gone. In God's hands." The hard lines around Angela's eyes had softened.

From then on, Angela stopped saying 'Me no can see'. She began listening to her favorite operas and chatted briefly with her grandchildren. On one of my visits, little Frankie was on her lap. "Mimi," he whispered. "Your eyes are beautiful. I wish you could see me."

Angela gently patted Frankie's cheeks and cupped his chin with her fingers. "Bambino, I see you from inside. You always part of me. *Ti amo.*"

"I love you too. You used to be sad. Now you're happier, even smile."

Angela pulled a lollipop out of her pocket of her robe, gave it to him, and kissed him on the forehead.

The morning before her surgery, Maria took her mother to the beauty shop for a haircut and set. Soft gray curls framed her round face. "I want to talk," she told Maria and me when I visited later that day.

We sat around their kitchen table.

"*Ti Amo*, Maria. You good daughter. What happens God's will. No longer want to burden you. Do what you think best if things don't turn out."

Tears filled Maria's eyes.

Angela turned toward me. "Put me in school for blind if operation go wrong, Lois. Maria has own life to live."

Maria replied, "I'll always be there for you, Ma. We'll work it out somehow." She wrapped her arms around Angela.

I thought how far this family had come in the last month. "There will be answers," I said.

The next day, Angela woke up early and asked Maria to help her dress in the red suit she'd always loved. The operation was routine, and Angela returned home the next day, white gauze patches taped over her eyes. She remained serene, rocking back and forth in her chair, her rosary beads in her hand. "I say twenty-five Hail Marys and Our Fathers last night," she told me. "Father Anthony is coming later for communion."

"I know how much he comforts you."

"I ready. We know soon, good or bad," she told me.

The day the bandages were to be removed at the doctor's office, Angela again wore her red suit. "For good luck," she said.

Maria reported that Dr. Guthrie untaped the eyes patches with care. With her rosary beads in her hands and praying the Hail Mary, Angela slowly opened her eyes. "A little light but gray too. Maybe get better?" She turned toward Maria.

Dr. Guthrie was optimistic yet warned the vision could deteriorate.

When I visited two weeks later, Frankie opened the door for me. "Mimi's in her room," he said.

I paused at the bedroom door, surprised to see Angela in bed with Maria sitting at her side.

Angela moaned, sobbed, and then whispered, "It dark. No different."

Maria hugged Angela and wept into her shoulder. Angela put her hands on Maria's head, gently combed through her hair with her strong fingers, and murmured, "We be all right, Maria. It meant to be. I go to special school to learn to live blind."

I waited a few seconds to center myself before I walked into the room.

"It's the nurse, Mama," Maria said.

Angela raised her head and gestured to me. "Come, sit, more work for us to do."

NURSING: IT'S WHAT I DO

*As a nurse, we have the opportunity to heal the heart, mind, soul,
and body of our patients. They may forget your name, but they
will never forget how you made them feel.*

Maya Angelou

Larry had just been home from the hospital for a week
recovering from injuries from a motorcycle accident. Fractured
femur, ruptured spleen, and multiple abrasions. His parents were
caring for him in their home, and I was his visiting nurse. "I'm
through with the hard part," he told me yesterday.

That was yesterday. This morning, his mother called the office
to let me know Larry had been rushed to the emergency room last
night. He died there three hours later.

Damn it, Larry shouldn't have died. He was only twenty-six,
the same age as I.

"We don't know what happened," his mother said. "We heard
a scream. I rushed into the bedroom and found him lying on the
floor." Her voice choked.

After I hung up the phone, I tried to make sense of his death.
Tears ran down my cheeks. *Why did I ever become nurse? Was I
really helping anyone get well?*

I went to the restroom, splashed water on my face, and dried
my eyes. Then I phoned my other clients to schedule the rest of
my visits.

Caitlyn, another young patient in her twenties, was first on my
list. Two years ago, she'd been diagnosed with Stage IV
lymphoma. She lived alone in a small house in a middle-class

neighborhood. Her faithful companion was an eight-year-old Irish Setter, who rarely left her side.

Last month, she'd been discharged from the hospital after completing IV antibiotic therapy to treat an infected PICC line. We'd agreed that today would be my last visit. "Unless you need me again once your chemotherapy is restarted," I said.

Caitlyn sat in her living room recliner looking more robust than I'd ever seen her. She'd gained several pounds since my first visit and was wearing make-up for a change. A Chicago Cubs baseball cap covered her bald head.

She gave me a quick wave and then resumed petting her dog that lay by her side. As usual, she acted strong and stoic but flat and emotionally detached while I completed the physical assessment. From the beginning, I'd felt resistance from her, an empty friendliness like a smiling porcelain doll too fragile to touch. Could I have done more to improve our relationship, probed beyond her typical monosyllabic answers? I knew little about her personal life or how she felt about having cancer, but there was no time to work on that now. I felt uncertain how well she would manage on her own but was grateful that the list of community resources I'd given her sat on her coffee table.

After reviewing her discharge instructions, I asked, "Do you have any questions?"

"No questions, Lois. But I wrote this letter to you. Don't open it now. Wait till you get home." She shoved an envelope in my hand.

I looked at the monogrammed stationery and quickly slipped it in my pocket. "Thank you, Caitlyn. Good luck." I started to hug her, but she gently pushed me away.

"Here comes my neighbor up the sidewalk. I'm paying her to help me get a shower every day and cook a few meals. Now don't call a social worker or chaplain on me. And don't get mushy either." Caitlyn's voice cracked. She looked away and instantly regained her composure and then signaled her neighbor to come in the back door while she shooed me out the front door with the wave of her hand.

I turned around, intending to walk back into her living room but changed my mind at the last minute. No time for indecision. Robert was next on my home visit list.

I drove to his apartment and found him sitting on his living room sofa staring at the CNN news on his television. He was in mild respiratory distress.

"You need your medicine. Try to relax, take some deep breaths." I grabbed his inhaler from the end table and handed it to him. After a couple puffs, his breathing returned to normal. He'd been dealing with chronic emphysema for years.

Recently, Robert received an additional diagnosis, metastatic lung cancer and just yesterday agreed to enroll in the in-home hospice program, so this would be my last visit. His only daughter was eight months pregnant and scheduled to deliver her baby next month. "I want to live to see the baby and maybe go to his baptism. It's gonna be a boy and they're naming him Robert after me. And I need to be sure my wife is okay, make certain she understands how to manage our finances organized before I ...." His voice became raspy.

"Your strong will and the hospice workers will help you," I said, hoping he'd achieve his goals, but I wasn't sure. For Robert, the line between life and death could be a mere thread.

He held out his hand. I put both my hands over his and said goodbye,

***

The day had been hectic; two new admissions and a distraught wife threatening to abandon her husband with Stage Two Alzheimer's Disease. I ended up working two hours overtime. *Why hadn't I dropped out of nursing school and gotten an easier job?* I arrived home tired and discouraged.

I set my nursing bag on the kitchen chair and told my husband, "I'm leaving nursing." When I stuffed my hands in my pockets to pull out my pens, a paper crinkled, Caitlyn's letter. I tore the envelope open.

Dear Lois,

Thank you for walking along my path these past weeks. From the moment I saw you, something pulled at me to get to know you. I regret that I never did. You don't know it, but you saved my life. Your life force pulled at mine and just wouldn't let it go.

I didn't want to live. I have a miserable lonely life. My dad abused me. I've been raped and robbed, assaulted at every turn. I don't trust anyone or anything.

I tried to push you away, but I couldn't. You were there, your presence held me strong.

Through all my misery I can still recognize a gentle smile and a kind heart, and for these things I am grateful. Thank you for looking beyond the patient and seeing the person behind my eyes, for reaching out to me and never expecting anything in return, for your generous and quiet compassion.

May God continue to bless you.

Peace,
Caitlyn

My eyes filled with tears. "I never knew she even cared," I told my husband. "Maybe I give more than I think. Maybe I have what it takes to be a nurse after all."

At that moment, I saw my career in a new light. Never before had it occurred to me that nursing allowed me to enter another's sacred space, sometimes when I didn't even know it. Caitlyn made me realize that my life energy can heal someone and that by giving, I receive.

***

As the years passed, I became even more convinced that nursing is a divine way to connect to others, to walk their path. To learn about them, about myself, about life.

Nursing, a sacred privilege, a crash course on living, a primer on dying.

Nursing. It's what I do.

FACING THE FEAR

Nothing in life is to be feared. It is only to be understood.
Marie Curie

I walked up the steps to Dominic's small ranch home concerned that I wouldn't be able to help him. His 75th birthday was last week. Several years ago, he had been diagnosed with slowly progressing macular degeneration, which forced him to give up his driver's license. His primary physician referred him to our home care agency to assess his cardiac and pulmonary status after a shortness of breath episode that resulted in a bathroom fall and a trip to the hospital's emergency room. There, he was diagnosed with aortic stenosis and referred to Dr. James, a cardiac surgeon. Adamantly opposed to heart surgery, he refused to make an appointment with the new doctor.

I found the house key Dominic often left for me under the pot of geraniums by the porch railing. When I opened the door, he was sitting at his small kitchen table. His hair was disheveled and his eyelids puffy. After his wife's death two years ago, Dominic had become a loner, estranged from his family and friends.

"I don't know why you keep coming. Why do you care what happens to me?" he asked.

I touched his shoulder and said, "Can we talk a bit about your heart?"

"Not today. Just do what you have to do. You've already explained a lot to me.

"All right. Next time. I'm here for you, but I hope you make the appointment with Dr. James soon. Is there anyone you can talk with about this, someone you trust, who you can confide in?"

"No, but would you find out more details about the surgery before I call the doctor? I've thought a lot about what you said, that leaving the problem go will damage my heart so much that I won't be able to live here alone anymore, and I am more tired and short of breath. I wish I could talk to my wife but....." Tears filled his eyes.

"I'll tell you what," I said. "I get you more details if you promise to make the appointment."

He nodded. "I know I've been slow, but I promise."

"Good," I answered. "Now let me check you out."

As I took Dominic's blood pressure and listened to his lungs, I thought of Helen Marks, a patient I met early in my nursing career. The downcast dark brown eyes, the furrowed brow, and the sad affect were the same.

***

Helen was blind and in her mid-forties. Her blindness was due to severe retinal damage, a complication of her premature birth. Our home health agency was called when she fell and cracked her pelvis. Her physician wanted her to be admitted to a nursing home for rehabilitation and muscle strengthening and then enrolled in a program for the visually impaired. She refused to do either and instead insisted on returning to her elderly mother's family home.

I remembered the day I visited the family for the first time and met Helen's mother, Dorothy.

"I don't know what to do with Helen anymore," she said with tears in her eyes. "She won't do anything for herself, even demands I feed her." She rubbed her hip. "My back's killing me from all the lifting."

"It's hard to care for an adult child. We'll find ways to make it easier. Take one step at a time." I took her hand and squeezed it.

"Helen's always been a good daughter. Always made me laugh and had a twinkle in her eyes even though she couldn't see. Now those eyes just stare into space."

"She sounds depressed."

"Yes, Dr. Phillips has prescribed pain pills and wants her to get up and walk a few steps, but she won't."

I fingered the stethoscope around my neck. "Let's go into the bedroom and see Helen now."

Helen was a thin pale woman with short curly auburn hair, who was lying flat on her back and staring into space. I took her hand and introduced myself.

She murmured, "Hello," and responded to my questions with monosyllabic answers.

I learned she had fallen getting out of bed and was afraid to try again. She accepted a physical therapy referral but refused to let me help her get up to walk. After deliberation, she and Dorothy agreed to a referral for a home health aide and social worker. I contacted her physician, who increased the dosage of her anti-depressant.

Over the next two weeks, I learned Helen rarely left the house since her high school graduation from a special school for the disabled. Since that time, she'd lived at home and remained dependent on her mother for her basic needs. In talking more with Dorothy, I saw how much Dorothy enjoyed taking care of Helen, which only fostered her daughter's dependence—an example of enabling and co-dependence often seen in families with disabled or chronically ill members.

One day, Marianne, the social worker phoned me. "Dorothy and Helen are both starting to understand that Helen is able to be more independent. I think there's a slim chance she'll enroll in the program for the visually impaired."

I took a deep breath. "The physical therapist has been working with Helen. She's getting up on her own and walks around the house now. There's no need for the in-patient rehab anymore. I've been talking with them, too. Dorothy has been worried that there will be no one to care for Helen after she dies. She's close to 80."

Marianne sighed.

"Helen worries about her mother and was able to tell her that," I said. "It was a break-through for both of them. Now, Helen's asking me questions about the program and is more receptive to enrolling."

"We've made a lot of progress," the social worker said.

After discovering that Helen had always wanted a dog, I contacted 'Leader Dogs for the Blind' and shared information on that program with Helen. She listened intently but offered few comments.

The following week Marianne and I made a joint visit. The four of us sat around the family's kitchen table. With a quivering lip, Helen said, "All right, I'll do it. I'll try the school for the blind. Then, I want a seeing-eye dog."

"Remember that's another live-in program?" I said.

She nodded. "I'm scared though. See how my fingers shake, but I feel different now. Just talking to you two has helped."

There was a change in Helen's face. The hard lines between her eyes had softened.

Dorothy looked at us. "I prayed last night something like this would happen and it did. Thank you."

I reached over and squeezed her arm. "One step at a time," I said.

***

I made a return visit to Dominic two days later. After completing the physical assessment, I said, "It's time to talk about the operation."

He swallowed hard. "Did you check any other options for me?"

I nodded. "A newer technique is done at the university. It can be used for people like you who are thin. It's not very invasive. Just an inch or two incision in the upper part of your chest between the ribs. It's one of Dr. James' specialties."

He smiled, and his entire face brightened. "Talking to you helped me, gave me hope. Yesterday, I called an old friend, someone I used to work with, haven't seen him for years."

"What happened?" I asked.

"We chatted for a half-hour. He's taking me to the doctor's appointment. I made it for next Thursday at one o'clock. He'll take me to the hospital if I need surgery and be there the day of the operation. I'm taking one step at a time."

A single tear ran down his cheek. I brushed it away.

WATERCOLORS IN THE RAIN

This is courage to bear unflinchingly what heaven sends.
Euripides

Sheets of rain pummeled the windshield as I parked my car in Harry Goldman's driveway. I grabbed my nursing bag and raced up the long winding sidewalk to his house, a large two-story colonial on a five-acre lot in an affluent suburb.

"It's Lois, your nurse," I said through the open screen door.

"I don't need a nurse," a man's crackly voice yelled. "Go away. Just let me be!"

I stood on the porch as the rain beat against the roof above me. Should I go back and tell my home health agency supervisor the client refused care? The patient, a seventy-nine year old man who'd had a right-sided stroke after abdominal surgery, needed help. He'd spent three weeks at a rehab center before coming home. Our agency would provide nursing, physical and occupational therapy, and social work services.

A home health aide dressed in a polyester white uniform appeared. The voice from inside the house continued, "I told you not to answer it, Lydia."

I flicked the water off my jacket and motioned Lydia outside.

"He's angry and depressed. Talks about dying. I haven't been able to get him out of bed since he came home yesterday," she reported.

"Anything else?"

"He was a wealthy businessman with several auto engine patents. Owns a small plant in the city and worked in the office there till five years ago. He's Jewish."

"Who lives with him now?"

"Two live-ins and I rotate. His wife died last year. Supposedly they didn't get along, but he's elevated her to sainthood since. He misses her. The house is big, but he only lives in two rooms."

Mr. Goldman's voice interrupted us, "Lydia, come help me. I'm trying to eat breakfast."

"I'll be right in," she said,

"Tell the nurse to go away."

Lydia persuaded him to relent. "Just for today, mind you,"

***

I walked into the bedroom. Mr. Goldman, dressed in beige pajamas, food drippings on the collar, lay propped up in a hospital bed. His gaunt face and thin frame accentuated his gray mustache and pale skin color. Floor-to-ceiling shelves filled with books lined one entire wall of the room. I glanced at the titles and saw many philosophers' names—Einstein, Swedenborg, and St. Thomas Aquinas. Watercolor landscapes and hand-drawn portraits of Albert Einstein hung on the opposite wall.

He looked up at me. "This damned stroke. I'm not trying to be difficult. I just don't want a nurse. I never wanted the surgery to start with."

"It's hard not to be able to do what you want."

"How would you know?"

"You're right. I don't really know."

He smirked. "I'm sick of exercises. Why should I learn to walk better? I have money, enough to pay for people to care for me. That's what money's for."

He squeezed the yellow exercise ball in his hand and threw it on the floor. Lydia quickly picked it up and put it on his bedside table.

"You were getting up and walking in rehab," I said.

"That was then. I just wanted to get well enough to go home. I want to die here," he said in a flat voice. He tried to make a fist with of his right hand. "I still can't do my watercolors."

"You did all these?" I asked, pointing to the portrait-filled walls.

He nodded as tears filled his eyes.

I rubbed his shoulders. His back muscles softened.

I fingered the stethoscope around my neck. "Can I check you over?" I asked.

"Whatever."

I listened to his lung sounds, then finished the rest of the physical assessment. He was alert and oriented with right-sided weakness, particularly his arm. I looked at the wheelchair by his bedside and nodded to Lydia.

"He won't," she mouthed.

"Would you sit in the wheelchair while we change your bed?" I asked Mr. Goldman.

"No need," he answered.

I pointed to the coffee stains on his sheets.

He nodded grudgingly. "Only for a minute."

***

On my visit three weeks later, Mr. Goldman was dressed, sitting in a chair looking at a photograph. He showed it to me and smiled. "My grandson, Adam's bar mitzvah is next month. He's a good boy. I need to be there for him. My grandfather was there for me until..." He cleared his throat and looked up to find my eyes. "He died in Auschwitz."

He straightened his shoulders. "Back to the stroke. I told the physical therapist to work me hard. I can walk across the room now."

At the case conference, the physical therapist concurred. "He's improving. He can walk twenty feet with his quad cane."

"He's still depressed," the social worker said. "The anti-depressants help, but he's anxious and has much unresolved grief about losing his wife. He just started opening up.

"I've had a breakthrough," I added. "Lydia and I have been reading to him from an Einstein book. A couple quotes got to him. Like 'Anger only dwells in the bosom of fools' and 'In the middle of difficulty lies opportunity.' He used his padded pencil to copy them into a journal and then started teaching his grandson how to draw animals. We're moving in the right direction."

***

The following week Mr. Goldman began to telephone the agency's on-call evening nurse with vague complaints of not feeling well. He refused a nursing visit, because the aide was there, but he wanted the nurse to talk with him.

I mentioned the problem to Lydia.

"He insists. I try to stop him from calling, but he has a stubborn streak. Gets what he wants."

"We'll let it go. The agency's okay with the calls for now."

On my next visit, Mr. Goldman ran his hand over his forehead and explained, "I'm looking for a connection to life. At night I panic I'll have another stroke."

"Do you tell Lydia?"

"No. Lydia and the other aides are fine. But there's something in the nurse's voice that's different, makes me feel protected."

I remembered the softness in the nurse's voice the night my mother died.

"I was a workaholic," he said. "Work gave me purpose. I'm useless now."

"Your courage is an example to Adam, Lydia, and me."

"I gave what I could to my children and the world, the patents, the money to charity, tutoring adults in reading. Einstein said service is better than power. Nursing is service too, isn't it?"

"Yes." My voice cracked.

"I wish I could have done more for my people."

"How so?"

"I grew up in Warsaw before the war. My family, my mother, my sisters...all lost...the camps...the Holocaust. I was the only one who got out. Some rabbi in New York did it... can't talk about it. It hurts too much." Tears came to his eyes. He turned his chair away from me and took a handkerchief from his pocket.

"Another time?"

He nodded. "My feelings are either dead or overwhelming. I like it better when they're dead."

"Even when we feel dead, embers burn underneath."

He turned his chair back toward me. "I'm waiting for them to burn out. At night they flare up."

I took his hand.

"Nights can be harder, because there's less going on."

"Maybe that's why I call the agency then, but I didn't call last night. I'm not religious, but I find comfort in the philosophies of the different faiths. Last night I reread the Bible verses about 'the lilies of the fields.' I've always liked it."

He pointed to a watercolor on the wall. "I painted that meadow of anemones. Some scholars say it was anemones that really grew in the lily field Matthew wrote about."

I looked again at the pink, blue, and lilac blossoms. "It's beautiful."

"The lily field passage helps me believe God will take care of me, like the anemones. And that I don't have to worry about tomorrow. Each day is a gift and a challenge unto itself."

I squeezed his hand. "You're going to be all right. Your courage, your character, your wisdom. No one can take that from you."

***

On the day of my last visit, there had been an early morning rain. But as I parked in his driveway, the sun was shining through the clouds. I felt whimsical walking up his winding sidewalk. He answered the door and welcomed me in.

After I reviewed his discharge instructions, Mr. Goldman handed me a small watercolor of Albert Einstein. Underneath, in shaky handwriting, he had written his name and *Without a sense of wonder, life is empty.* "What you've done for me is too much to talk about, so I've drawn this for you."

I smoothed his cheeks with the backs of my fingers. "Thank you. I'll keep it always."

And I have. It sits on my desk, and each time it rains, I remember the man who first told me to go away but then welcomed me into his heart.

BENEATH THE VENEER

You treat a disease, you win or you lose. You treat a person, I guarantee you win, no matter what the outcome.

Patch Adams.

The phone call from the Maxwell's son came into the home health agency late one afternoon. "Mom's in the hospital. She had a mild heart attack Monday night."

"And your dad was the one we were worried about." I shook my head. "So unexpected. She was such a caregiver. She wanted to do it all, even seemed to thrive on it."

"I know. Never let Lisa or me help. Not that we often asked. We're transferring Dad to a nursing home till she gets better. We never dreamed he was so much work." His voice choked.

***

On my first home visit several months ago, Mr. Maxwell lay propped on pillows in a hospital bed in the middle of family's small living room. A trapeze hung over the head of the bed. A glass of water and a half-finished jigsaw puzzle sat on his bedside table. He'd already been bedridden for two years. A ruptured cerebral aneurysm and complications from Type 2 diabetes left him with urinary incontinence, left sided paralysis, and a right foot amputation. His dark wavy hair, small physique, and bright brown eyes made him look younger than his fifty-nine years.

I was one of the home health care nurses assigned to make monthly supervisory visits and change his Foley catheter as needed. From the beginning, I was impressed by Mrs. Maxwell's commitment to her husband's care and her indestructible attitude. She turned him frequently to keep his skin free from pressure sores and used a Hoyer Lift to transfer him into his wheelchair every day. Always upbeat, often laughing or telling funny stories, she kept Mr. Maxwell entertained. She was consistently well groomed, energetic, fit and trim. Often, the aroma from freshly baked cookies drifted in from the kitchen. "I always use a sugar substitute," she told me.

Alone with her in the kitchen one day, I asked, "Do your children give you a hand?" We sat at the table reviewing her emergency plan. She smiled. "No need for that. They have busy lives, jobs, young children. "

"Caring for Mike is a heavy load. A lot of work, day in and day out. It can take a toll."

"I enjoy it. With the kids grown, what else would I do? I've always been a homemaker, never liked going out much. Mike deserves the best. He's always worked hard, and he appreciates what I do for him. He sleeps through the night, so I get my eight hours in, too. My neighbor, we've been friends for years, stays with him when I go grocery shopping."

She declined my offers for blood pressure checks, home health aide services, and a referral to a social worker or caregiver's support group. "I see my doctor every January for a physical. Everything's fine. I haven't the time or interest in a support group. I went to one a long time ago. All people did there was complain."

The nursing visits fell into an easy routine. My referral suggestions for respite help were infrequent. Mrs. Maxwell appeared happy and content. Mr. Maxwell's condition remained stable. "She doesn't miss a beat taking care of me," he said.

***

Now both Mr. and Mrs. Maxwell were part of my patient load. When I arrived on that first return visit, Mrs. Maxwell was sitting in a recliner chair. Mr. M was lying in his living room hospital bed. A home health aide was in the bathroom organizing the supplies to bathe him after I left.

Mr. Maxwell shook his head. "You don't know how wonderful it is to be home. I never appreciated all Kathy did until

I lost it. He turned to his wife. "You're never doing it all by yourself again."

She stifled a sob. "I hate that this happened. I enjoy taking care of you."

He sighed. "We still have each other. That's more important than anything."

After I took her vital signs, Mrs. Maxwell smiled weakly. Her skin was pale; she'd lost some weight, but her prognosis was for a full recovery. Cardiac rehab would start next week.

"It's been a wake-up call, Lois. You were right, what you said a long time ago about getting help. The doctor said stress was part of the problem. Funny, I never felt stressed. I wanted to do it all by myself, but...." Her voice trailed off.

Mr. Maxwell turned his head. "It wasn't fair to her or the kids either. They missed seeing the real us. And understanding life's not always a bowl of cherries. And I learned the hard way how difficult it was to trust someone else to take care of me. The nursing home people do things differently, but somehow it all worked out. I may go back again to give her a break."

I swallowed hard. "You'll have the home health aide and a physical therapist three times a week plus a couple social work visits to talk about a long term care plan."

Mrs. Maxwell looked up. "I'll try the suggestions, even having the van pick me up and take me to cardiac rehab. I have no choice, really. I can't imagine anyone caring for Mike like I used to. I'm still not going to a support group. Hate that idea."

"What you're doing at home here is a good start. It helps Mike to know you're not going to be so overworked. If you don't take care of yourself, there won't be anyone to take care of him."

Mr. Maxwell spoke. "One good thing about all of this is that our son is coming by a couple times a week to help. His wife brings over frozen meals we can just heat up, their leftovers, I guess, but the food tastes good.

Mrs. Maxwell said, "Our daughter still finds it hard to see us this way. She did agree to drive me to the doctor's next week." Tears filled her eyes. "I feel so worthless."

I nodded. "Your whole life's been turned upside down. It's like starting from Square One again. People are here to help; they care about you both. It will take time."

***

Sometimes, caregiver burden isn't recognized until it is too late. Attention to the caregiver's physical and mental health is as important as caring for the client. With the Maxwell's, the caregiver stress was hidden.

My work with the M family taught me that, especially if there's only one family caregiver, I need to dig beneath the veneer of *Everything's all right. I'm managing fine.* Caregiver needs and referral options should regularly be explored in depth—the positives, the negatives and the rationale behind them. Once that's done though, nurses must respect the client/family decision and work within those parameters.

THE LAST DANCE

When I die, I'm going to dance first in all the galaxies...
I'm gonna play and dance and sing.

Elisabeth Kubler-Ross.

Ella, fifty-two years old and dying, sat propped in her hospital bed. She looked frail and vulnerable; her big brown eyes begging for help.

***

Ella, a widowed housewife with congestive heart failure, had a stroke two months ago. As the visiting nurse assigned to her rehab team, I monitored her vital signs and taught her about her medications and ways to conserve energy. An anti-depressant lessened her melancholy. The physical therapist and I noted slow, steady progress in her endurance.

A heart attack erased those gains and gave her a new diagnosis, cardiomyopathy. "We need to begin palliative care," the doctor said.

"Not yet," I replied. "Ella just told me her son, Terry, is getting married. Her last wish is to dance at his wedding."

The physician temporarily increased Ella's heart medication to the maximum dose. The physical therapist and I worked on her balance. Soon she could stand alone for short periods and take small steps to compensate for her weakened right leg. Still, she became exhausted and short of breath in minutes.

In time, her activity tolerance improved. I practiced slow dancing with her, both of us wearing sturdy tennis shoes.

"I can't wear these clunkers to Terry's wedding," she said. I found dressy flats in her closet. "I hate this illness," she cried when her feet were too swollen to put them on. Terry's fiancé, Lainey, bought her two new pairs.

Ella laughed when she saw the shoes. "There's a blue garter in my sock drawer I want you to have, Lainey. I wore it on my wedding day." Lainey hugged Ella and put the garter around her wrist. Tears filled my eyes.

Finding a dress for the wedding was the next project. "I'd like something in soft pink," she said. Her friend came by with six different styles. Ella chose a long satiny one.

***

As time went on, Ella's body became frailer but her spirit stronger. The morning of the wedding, a beautician came to the home and added golden highlights to her brown hair, styled it in an upsweep, and manicured her nails, painting them pink to match the dress.

Exhausted from her efforts, Ella fell asleep.

Nurses' aides woke her an hour later to dress her. Soon, weak and short of breath, she laid down again. We prayed she'd make it through the day.

Getting her to the car in her wheelchair was easy; transferring her into the front seat was difficult. In a last burst of effort, she stood, bracing herself on her walker, and slid into the passenger's seat. She wanted to get to the church early, so she could be seated before the other guests arrived.

Tears ran down her face during the ceremony. When the service ended, many friends approached to offer congratulations. We encouraged them to move on; Ella's lips were turning blue, her breathing shallow and rapid. Medication relaxed her. We transferred her by wheelchair into the reception hall where she soon fell asleep on a sofa. She missed dinner. We woke her when the wedding cake was to be cut.

Everyone stood as she entered the room in her wheelchair. Sobbing, Ella whispered, "Thank you." Terry wheeled her in front of the table with the wedding cake. After the newlyweds cut the cake and fed each other, Terry handed his mother a piece. She ate it with shaking hands and laughed when she got icing on her face. Lainey wiped it off with a napkin.

The dancing started when the band played, *You Light up my Life.* Terry helped Ella stand, holding her gently in his arms. They danced cheek-to-cheek, moving in time to the music, in spite of Ella's dragging right foot. Afterwards, Terry led her back to her chair. A smile on her face, Ella sat and watched as more dancers took to the floor. She cheered her son when he removed the garter from Lainey's thigh.

After Ella's niece caught the bouquet of flowers Lainey threw into the crowd of single women, the nurses' aides took Ella home. "God bless you," she mouthed as her wheelchair rolled out the door.

***

Ella lived just long enough to see the wedding photos.

THINGS MONEY CAN'T BUY

After a certain point, money is meaningless. It ceases to be the goal. The game is what counts.

Aristotle Onassis

Monday morning would be hectic. Two new referrals plus my regular home visits. My first client, an 80-year-old widow, Matilda Casper, was staying with her daughter while she recovered from knee surgery.

Sunlight streamed through Matilda's bedroom window against an upholstered beige wingback chair. A twin bed, dresser, and nightstand stood against the far wall.

Matilda, a heavy-set woman wearing a mauve terrycloth robe, sat in a manual wheelchair with a pink hand-knit afghan across her knees. The sparkle in her azure blue eyes belied the fact that she'd just had major surgery to repair a crushed kneecap.

I introduced myself and put my hand on her shoulder. "How does it feel to be out of the rehab center?"

Matilda covered my hand with her pudgy fingers. "Tired, honey, but ready to work."

"You'll be busy. The physical therapist will visit three days a week and set up an exercise program."

Matilda sat up straighter in her wheelchair. "That's what I want. To get back home to my old life."

I smiled. "You have a good attitude. It'll help."

She pointed to a photograph on her dresser. "Those are my kids—four of 'em. The two in the middle live in California. Elaine and Denise live here in town."

"You have family around then."

"Yep, I'm lucky that way. The grandkids visit a lot."

I checked Matilda's balance, ability to rise from a chair, and leg strength and flexing capability. Both legs were weak, and the affected knee was very stiff, but the muscles in her upper extremities remained solid.

***

My next visit was to Nathan Castleman, a 78-year-old, who was lying in bed watching television as I entered the bedroom of his 4,500 square foot ranch home.

"Good morning, Mr. Castleman." I extended my hand toward his, noting his gaunt unshaven face, thinning gray hair, and the hearing aid in his left ear. His silk maroon bathrobe had coffee stains on the lapel and dandruff on the back collar. An electric wheelchair occupied one corner of the room.

Nathan kept his eyes on the *Today* show. "Not much good about it," he bellowed.

His speech was not slow and halting like some patients with Parkinson's, but severe tremors in his left hand and the slow way he moved his arms and legs could be a problem. His muscles were rigid when he changed positions to sit or stand, and he walked with a shuffling unsteady gait and displayed significant balance problems.

He's depressed, I thought, making a note to notify his physician. "Mind if I check you out? Ask you a few questions?" I sat down on the chair by his bed.

"Do what you want. I'm going to cancel your agency after today." He pointed to a plaque on the wall over to the head of his bed. "You don't recognize my name?"

"Oh, no. I didn't at first. Of course, *Castleman's Tool and Die* on Second Street."

He turned toward me. "That's me. I don't need rehab. I have lots of money and can afford to pay for anything I want. That includes someone to push me around in a chair, get me where I want to go, carry me if needed. Rehab is for the birds."

"Why did you let me come then?"

"Doc says he'll dump me if I don't try rehab. I slipped getting out of the shower last week. Bruised my hip and sprained my back but nothing's broken. No big deal."

"But a good reason for me and a physical therapist to be here. It's hard not to be able to walk."

He squeezed his left hand into a tight ball. "I have thought about that. A lot. I'll be fine. I'm seventy-eight, have this damn Parkinson's, but I can still think. Godammit, I'm a multimillionaire, not a weakling."

"For sure, not a weakling. Otherwise, you wouldn't be as successful as you are."

"Till last week, I worked half days in the office. A chauffeur drove me every morning; now he'll take me in a wheelchair; I'll buy a van with a lift." He fingered the remote control. "I'm not going to live forever. Why not make the rest of my life easy?"

I pulled my chair up closer to the bed and pressed a wrinkle from his sheet. "Strengthening your muscles will help you walk better and stay independent. If you don't rehab those muscles now, you'll lose the function. It won't be easy to get your strength back later. Give it your best effort for three weeks. Then decide."

Nathan frowned. "You sound like Dr. Potter. Think you know what's best for me. But all right. At least my son doesn't come to the house begging for money. He only visits me in my office."

"That must be hard."

He turned his face to the wall. "Enough talking. I'm tired."

The following week, I spoke with Mr. Castleman's aide, Ken. "Dr. Potter agrees Nathan's depressed but says to let him move at his own pace. Push him but not too hard. He's not ordering antidepressants, partly because Nathan doesn't believe in them."

Ken fingered the pen in his pocket. "Nate wouldn't take antidepressants if prescribed. He moves around in the electric wheelchair and refuses to do his range of motion exercises or use his walker."

I nodded. "He's a challenging patient. Thanks for updating me.

***

Two days later I made a shared home visit with Shelly, the physical therapist. When Nathan asked to end the session after fifteen minutes, she said to him, "Take a rest. Then, let's finish these exercises we started."

Nathan turned around in his electric wheelchair to face me. "I've finished everything in my life worth finishing. In case she doesn't know, I pay for what I need."

My eyes met his steely brown ones. "Some things you just can't buy," I said.

"There's nothing in this world worth having that can't be bought."

"Let's talk a bit about that idea." My words echoed against the walls. Nathan was wheeling himself out of the room.

Ken ran his fingers through his hair. "He's been uncooperative. Complains about the therapy every day."

"It can take a while for patients to adapt to the routine. Let's give him more time."

***

I left Nathan's house to visit Matilda. Why couldn't Nathan be more like her? If only he would follow Shelly's treatment plan like Matilda had, he might be up and about with his walker. Matilda now walked with a quad cane.

Matilda moved her arms up and down as she talked with me. "I can't wait to get home. My big house is waiting for me. Lived there fifty-three years, raised the kids there, and stayed on after George died. I miss my kitchen and can still bake the best pies in the world."

"If you go home too soon, you could have a setback."

"So much for 'ifs.' They don't get you anywhere. I learned that when I was stopped at a red light and the drunk driver slammed into me and crushed my knee. If I had only left the house five minutes earlier. If this, if that. All hogwash excuses. Let's practice stair walking."

I remembered Shelly's directions. "Put your good foot up first going up the stairs and your bad foot first coming down. A good way to remember is that the good go first to heaven and the bad go first to Hell."

"Shelly says once I master steps, I can go home."

"When you do go home, I'd recommend a lifeline to alert someone that you need help if you fall or have an emergency?"

She laughed. "You nurses always think ahead."

Two weeks later Ken phoned the agency. "Nathan fell. He didn't call me, got up on his own and seems okay but...."

I added his name to my afternoon schedule. He was sitting in his wheelchair when I arrived. "I slid out of the chair and used the footstool to get up. By myself!"

I noted no injuries from his fall; but, after that day, Nathan began to follow the therapist's directions. Three weeks later, his balance and lower leg strength had improved enough that he could use a walker to ambulate and get out of a chair. "How am I doing?" he asked.

"Wonderful. There's been a big difference from the day you were admitted."

"Shelly wants me to work on stair climbing, but I don't want to. I rarely go down to the basement."

"Steps can be in the most unexpected places."

Nathan took his hearing aid out and put it in his pocket. He looked away.

I pointed to his pocket and motioned to his ear.

Nathan fingered his hearing aid and inserted it back in his ear. "In case you don't know, I decide what I need to learn, not you." Yet he held onto the basement banister and placed his right leg on the step. "You don't know what it's like to be in my shoes."

"Tell me," I said.

Nathan took a deep breath. "I'm a failure as a father. When my son used to visit, he'd always ask for money, needed this and that. Never worked a full day in his life, and he's forty-nine. I have more cash than I'll ever spend, and it was simpler to hand the money over to him. No arguments. No fuss. He hasn't visited since I stopped working."

I swallowed hard. "It can feel good to give the kids what they want, but it doesn't make for good character building. And you can't buy love."

"I'm just figuring that out." Nathan took a deep breath. "I want to apologize for the way I talked to you in the beginning. It's been a tough year for me."

"How so?"

Nathan sighed. "Since Frances died, I've been a mess. She kept me on a straight course. Never thought I'd miss her. We fought so much, mostly over little things."

"I can understand that."

"Frances died of an aneurysm. She was fine when we went to bed. At four a.m., she was dead. Finding her on that hard tile bathroom floor was the worst kind of nightmare. I uh..." He wiped his rheumy eyes with his shirtsleeve. "We don't know what we have until we lose it. A good woman's one thing money can't buy. My son's love is another. Add doing things for myself to that list."

I swallowed hard. To think I had measured his progress against Matilda's, who had a supportive and caring family.

Nathan had to work through his grief and life losses in his own way and at his own pace. My job was to support him on his journey.

THE CRISIS

The patient decides when it's best to let go.
Jack Kevorkian

One afternoon, I picked up the home health care agency phone to hear the frightened voice of Peter Ramos. "My mother's dying. Can someone come?" His clipped words tumbled into my ear staccato-like fashion.

A new admission, a possible hospice referral. Taking a deep breath, I asked, "Do you need someone today or can you wait until morning?"

"She might not be here in the morning." His voice turned thick, husky.

"Give me your address and the physician's name. When I get the doctor's orders, I'll come." Two hours later, with end-of-life orders from the physician, I arrived at his house.

Unshaven, Peter Ramos, probably in his mid-forties, answered the door. His bloodshot eyes and rumpled cotton shirt told the story.

I placed my hand on his arm. "Let's talk before I see your mother."

He led me into the den and motioned for me to sit. "Thanks for coming so quickly. I never thought I'd need a nurse. I'm an EMT."

"Tell me what's been happening."

"Mother's seventy-four. Until a month ago, she was going to church and babysitting the grandkids." His voice quivered. "She lives with us." He pointed to a photo of Mrs. Ramos, a heavy-set smiling woman wearing a flowered dress. Tears filled his eyes.

I leaned forward. "This has to be hard. I'll do everything I can."

"I would do anything to save her, but there's nothing left to do." His voice cracked. "We haven't had enough time to prepare ourselves."

"It's hard when it happens so quickly," I said.

"We've been taking care of her around the clock since she came home. The rest of the family is in Mexico or they'd be here helping. One of us sits with her all the time. We don't want her to die alone or suffer."

"Have you signed a Do-Not-Resuscitate order?

He sighed. "Yes, and we've made funeral arrangements."

I looked at the DNR form he handed me and nodded. "Is she in pain or restless?"

"She seems calm and comfortable. She was on oral morphine and steroids until this morning. She can't swallow anymore. I've started the injections," he said.

"I can insert a small tube just under her skin for the morphine, so you won't need to poke her again."

He nodded. "Thank you. My sisters gave her tilia until this morning."

"Tilia?"

"The linden flower herb that acts as a sedative. The *yerbero*, the herbalist, recommended it."

"Any other herbs?"

"Not anymore."

"All right. Let's go see your mother now."

We entered the bedroom. Propped up on pillows and wearing a long-sleeved flannel nightgown, Mrs. Ramos lay in the middle of a double bed under a royal blue satin comforter. The sound of her raspy breaths filled the room.

Peter introduced me to his sisters, Theresa and Rosa, standing by their mother's bed. Both had pulled their long black hair into buns on the tops of their heads. Rosa, wearing a plaid housecoat with coffee-colored stains down the front, was applying compresses to her mother's forehead from a basin of warm water.

Theresa was praying the 'Hail Mary', her fingers moving rapidly over black rosary beads.

I assessed Mrs. Ramos. Her cold extremities, thready pulse, uneven breathing, and diminished reflexes told me the end was near. She appeared tranquil.

Theresa massaged her mother's arms and legs and pleaded, "Please live, Mama. Get well."

Rosa dried her mother's face with a towel. She pulled me aside. "Mama's slipping. She could open her eyes yesterday."

"She's very ill."

"The four humors were in better balance yesterday," Theresa said.

I remembered the Mexican belief that the forces of hot and cold as well as wet and dry needed to be in harmony for a person to be healthy. "What have you done for her?" I asked.

"We bathed her in warm water and keep her covered with blankets. It's not working. Maybe she got cold or maybe we are not praying enough."

"You're all doing a good job taking care of her."

Peter ran his fingers through his hair. "I hope it was right to bring her home."

I touched his arm. "Probably it's what she would have wanted."

He nodded. "Carlos, the *curandero*, sees Mother, too."

Theresa added, "Peter thinks Mama's dying. He doesn't believe in folk medicine. You probably don't either."

"The *curandero*, the faith healer, can help sometimes, but doctors can help, too. Your mother's very sick. We want to keep her comfortable."

Theresa's voice broke into a long sob. "I'm afraid her life is nearly over."

Tears filled both women's eyes. Rosa laid her head on her mother's chest.

I put my arm over her shoulder. "People die when it's the right time."

"That's what Carlos told me. Maybe Peter's right. Maybe Mama will soon be in Heaven." Theresa said.

"Why don't you sit around your mother's bed? Put your hand on her arms, legs, or face and take turns talking to her. Hearing's the last sense to go."

"Carlos said we should talk to her, too."

"I'll go in the other room and leave you all alone for a bit."

I walked to the kitchen and worked on my charting. When I returned to the bedroom, Mrs. Ramos looked peaceful; the children's tears had dried. Seeing me enter, Rosa asked, "The priest was here yesterday and gave her last rites, but how do we know if she has sin on her soul? I worry."

"I'll call the *curandero*," Peter suggested.

Carlos arrived an hour later. "Let's make a circle around her bed and pray."

Wiping her eyes with a tissue, Rosa asked, "Is she at peace?"

"Yes, your mother's at peace," Carlos whispered.

A sudden spasm crossed Mrs. Ramos' face as she took a deep breath, a breath that I knew was her last.

Tears ran down Peter and Theresa's cheeks. "She's gone," Rosa sobbed. Tears filled my eyes too, as I placed my stethoscope on her chest and pronounced her dead.

"You can stay with your mother for a while," I said.

"Yes, we need to be by ourselves," Peter said.

He put his arms around his sisters and wiped their tears from their faces. Carlos stood over them all, speaking in soft, soothing tones.

I gathered my supplies. "I'll notify the doctor. Is there anything else, calling the funeral home?"

"No, I know what to do."

He walked me to the door and grasped my hand in both of his. His fingers felt cold. "Thank you. I never realized a visiting nurse could help us so much."

"You're welcome. I'm glad to have met you and your family."

"Nurses. What a Godsend," he whispered.

THE OTHER CHEEK

To be wronged is nothing unless you continue to remember it.
Confucius

"Can you take a new referral?" my home health supervisor asked. "It's that priest, Father Dan, shot last month at St. Margaret's. He's being discharged from rehab tomorrow and needs teaching on colostomy care."

I grabbed my pen to write down his phone number. "I saw the news clips on TV. Shot by a crack addict."

"The bullet ripped his gut. He's going to his brother's to recuperate from the surgery."

***

The next morning I stocked my bag with handouts on colostomy care and the necessary supplies. I'd spent the night before worrying how to communicate with a priest. My uncle was a conservative Lutheran minister, and I'd always been in awe of clergy. Talk to the priest in a personal manner, look at his body! It was hard to imagine. I scheduled a late morning visit. When I walked into Father Dan's bedroom, he was still in pajamas.

I shook his hand. "How are you?"

"All right," he mumbled. "I slept like a baby last night. My own bed, I guess."

I looked at his steel gray eyes and blond curly hair. He appeared older and thinner than his TV photos. A chain with a gold cross hung around his neck. He hobbled over to get his robe from the chair. "I don't have pain anymore, but my muscles don't work right."

I learned that he was forty-nine and ran a food distribution and recreational program for the poor besides his parish duties. He talked easily about his past. "I was a maverick kid with lots of friends but no serious life focus. I breezed through the seminary, then was assigned to a suburban church. I felt useless there and nearly left the priesthood when the diocese transferred me to St. Margaret's. The church was dying. Reviving it gave my life meaning."

I relaxed, grateful he seemed sure of his spirituality, or so I thought. At least I wouldn't need to address spiritual problems. I said, "We'd better stop talking and get to work."

I checked his vital signs and listened to his lungs. The wound on his abdomen had become infected in the rehab center. We cleaned and measured the incision and then changed the dressing.

***

Over the next week, I learned more about Father Dan. "I ride a motorcycle, you know. Before I came to St. Margaret's, it and prayer were my only comforts."

"You must have been unhappy."

"And confused. St. Margaret's changed me. The inner city people gave me a purpose. I felt like I made a difference in their lives."

One day as we were organizing his supplies, tears came to his eyes. "I hate who I've become. I'll never be a good person again."

My heart jumped. "What do you mean?"

"I'm not sure there's a God out there. Maybe that's why I talk so much about my past and not what's going on now."

I took a deep breath, realizing I'd been wrong not to have addressed the spiritual aspects of his care and quickly changed my focus. "The shooting, did it shatter your faith?"

His eyes widened. "You're the first person to ask. And I've had a lot of visitors, many priests. Everyone assumes my religion will carry me through. They only want to talk about the police investigation, what's going on at the parish, or the violence on TV." He started to sob and looked directly at me. "Why did he shoot me? He didn't have to. I would have given him money."

"Tell me what happened."

"He barged in and pulled out a gun. Rudy was his name. Started screaming he needed crack. The next thing I knew, I was lying on a gurney in the hospital's emergency room."

"What a shock!"

Father Dan clenched his fists. "Rudy started coming to the church office last month. We'd talk. I thought he respected me."

"You trusted him then?"

"I did. He'd finished outpatient rehab and had stayed clean. Must've relapsed that very day." He pointed to his soiled dressing that I'd just removed from his wound. "He gave me this to remember him by. He's in jail now. His trial date isn't set yet, but I'll have to testify."

"I'm sorry you have to go through this."

"I used to think serving the poor was my life's mission. Now I'm not sure. I can't forgive him. I want to. I try to pray, but I can't." Father Dan picked up a Bible on his nightstand.

A lump formed in my throat. "Would you like me to read to you?"

He nodded. I chose the twenty-third psalm. He covered his face with his hands, then started to talk. "I wake up at night trembling. In my dream I'm beating him, sometimes to death. I'm afraid my anger will never go away. What should I do, leave the priesthood? I can't serve others feeling this angry." He hesitated, then whispered, 'Father, forgive them for they know not what they do.' I can't forgive."

I touched his arm. "Maybe when you work through this, you'll be able to serve the people better. Would you like to talk with our social worker?"

"No one can help me."

"Will you try it? It's common for victims of violent crimes to blame themselves."

"All right."

***

When I visited three weeks later, Father Dan had talked with the social worker several times. "She helped me understand how I have a physical wound and Rudy a mental one."

"Hmm, which is worse?"

"I don't know. But I'll take my life over his. He grew up in foster care. Lived in six different homes before he was eighteen. My pain's easier to heal. His will last his lifetime."

In a conversation two weeks later, Father Dan said, "I wrote him ten letters, ripped up the first nine. Mailed the last one yesterday. Told him I forgive him."

"That's a huge step forward," I said.

***

On my last visit, Father Dan greeted me with a smile. "The incision's almost healed. No more antibiotics. No more visits to the surgeon. He discharged me yesterday."

"You look happy."

"I preached on Sunday. After mass, I knelt at the altar and prayed for Rudy and myself. And later in the afternoon, Cardinal Anthony asked me develop a comprehensive project for the city's homeless. Housing, food, job training. I'm excited."

I took his hand. "You've found God again."

His grasp was strong. "Yes, I understand now He never left me."

THE TEACHER

The best teachers teach from the heart, not from the book.
Author unknown

The ringing cell phone startled me. My home health care nursing supervisor was on the line. "Lois, we got a new referral. Sounds complex. A sixty-year old woman who just finished treatment for a large blood clot in her leg. She also has multiple sclerosis and hasn't been out of bed for five months. She's supposed to be demanding and depressed. Can you see her tomorrow?"

"Of course," I replied. Clients with both physical and psychological issues had always intrigued me. Many of them gave me a blueprint on how I might live my life as an older person. Irma Higgins was no exception.

I pulled my car into her driveway the next morning. The two-story freshly painted colonial home was set back from the street. Maple trees and brightly colored peonies filled the yard.

Before I rang the bell, the door quickly sprung opened. "You must be the nurse. I'm Jim Higgins, Irma's husband. She's in there."

I walked into the small living room. Wooden shelves filled with books of various sizes and colors took up the entire space along one wall. Piles of children's books lay on the floor. Irma sat propped up in her hospital bed in the back corner of the room. She wore a white silky nightgown under a soft pink flannel bed jacket. Short gray hair framed her round face. As she looked at me, tears formed in the corners of her big brown eyes and slowly rolled down her cheeks.

"I didn't want you to come, but Dr. Trent insisted. He says I need help, that I can't stay in bed all the time. I wish I could hide under the covers like I did when I was a little girl. I don't want to get up at all anymore, ever." She was sobbing now.

I squeezed her hand. "I'm here to try to make things better for you. You're the boss though. We'll work out a plan together, one with your stamp of approval on it."

As I did my initial assessment, I noted that multiple sclerosis had made her legs flaccid and her back muscles weak. Irma looked at least fifty pounds overweight. The flannel bed jacket covered flabbiness in her upper arms. She told me she had been an elementary school teacher in her earlier years and described herself as 'someone from the old school', a taskmaster of sorts.

Irma's husband cared for her. She summoned him to her bedside with an old-fashioned cow bell. Jim spent hours every day cooking meals, washing clothes, emptying bedpans, and ironing sheets. She insisted on ironed white lightly starched sheets for her mattress and fresh flowers for her nightstand.

Many times I consoled her while she cried about her illness and the burden she was to her husband. "Would you let an aide get you washed up?" I said. "Caring for you is taking its toll on Jim. He never complains, but I know he gets awfully tired sometimes."

"Give, give, give. Why am I the one always having to make the adjustments?"

"I know it's hard. Deep down, though, you know everyone is making adjustments. Letting Jim off the hook for some of your care would be a big help to you both. If he gets sick, there would be no one to take his place."

In the end, she agreed to accept the aide on a two-week trial basis. "I want it done my way," she told me.

I reviewed Mrs. Higgins' care plan carefully with the nursing assistant. "I like having a woman bathe me," she told me later. "She's more careful and keeps the water warmer than Jim does. It's okay. I'm glad I made the change. Jim still does the bed bath on the weekends."

"Would you like to try to get in the shower and get washed up sitting on a special chair?" I asked her.

"No way" she yelled. "I've given in to you enough. Why did God do this to me anyway?" she shrieked. "I'm no good to anybody. I never would have thought I would need someone to give me a bath in bed."

This sad angry mindset was never apparent on Monday or Wednesday afternoons. Those days were "school days", days when her hospital bed was rolled up to a full sitting position, make up applied to her face, and horn-rimmed bifocal glasses on her nose. Every Monday and Wednesday, four second grade students came to her home for tutoring. All the students had problems with cognitive immaturity and short attention spans. Each child lived in the neighborhood, and the mothers provided transportation.

Jim put wooden chairs on each side of Irma's bed for the kids. A plate of chocolate chip cookies lay on her bedside stand. The warmth and caring she shared with those children was infectious. She saved her jolliness especially for them.

When the kids came in, Irma hugged each one and asked, "What special thing happened to you today?" Then, Mrs. Higgins gave each child crayons and pieces of brightly colored construction paper. "Draw a picture and write words to tell me about it," she said. Next she pulled books about the kid's drawings from her shelves.

"Read us the story, Mrs. Higgins," the children said in unison.

"We'll read together," she responded. And read together they did. I can still see the kid's little fingers following the lines on the page while listening to her instructions. "Sound it out now. Make the M sound. See, you got it right."

Soon all four children had pulled their chairs in closer to crowd around her bed before their class ended with cookies and milk.

After the children left, she'd be exhausted, yet she had enough energy to ring her bell. "Brush the cookie crumbs out of the bed," she demanded. I don't know why I keep tutoring. Working with the kids makes my muscles tense up. And such a mess afterwards. I should stop this nonsense."

I seized the opportunity to give her a reason to get out of bed. Getting up to shower didn't work, but maybe this would. "How about trying to sit up for your classes? The physical therapist can get us equipment to help you sit in your wheelchair. You can put the bedside table right in front of you. The kids will be so excited."

"No, I don't think so, Lois. It would be too hard, too much work."

"Just think about it," I replied. "See you next week."

I was surprised to find Mrs. Higgins smiling when I arrived the following Friday. "Maybe you're right about sitting up to tutor," she said. "Maybe I have another gift to give to the children. Something more important than reading. How to overcome immense handicaps. How to survive and make a difference in people's lives and have a positive attitude."

"Yes," I said. "You're so right. You can do this, I'm sure. Maybe, it's your mission, a special calling."

The therapist and Irma worked diligently for three weeks. When I arrived one day, she was sitting in her wheelchair.

"I wanted to surprise you," she said. "It's because of you that I am sitting here. And I can't believe how good it feels. I can only sit for five or ten minutes now, but every day it will get better. Maybe I'll even try to get in the shower soon."

Her endurance in the sitting position increased every day. In two weeks, she was ready to see the kids.

The children clamored all at once when they walked through the door. "Wow, Mrs. Higgins, you can sit now. You're getting better. You look more like our regular teacher now. Will we still get cookies? Why did you decide to sit in your wheelchair?"

Irma paused, waiting for them to quiet down. "We can study better this way," she said. "It's easier for us to write and follow the words in the book with our fingers. Sometimes if we have a problem, we have to work harder and that makes what we do more special. I've worked hard to do my exercises every day so I can sit in my wheelchair just like I want you to work hard on your reading every day."

"You're like us then. We have reading exercises, and you have arm and leg exercises."

"Yes," Irma smiled. "You have it in a nutshell."

I looked down at the little group and thought, *May I live my life with so much courage in the face of adversity, Irma. I'll never forget you.*

SMOKE TINGED GLASSES

The art of being wise is knowing what to overlook.
William James

Kathy, a nursing student at an inner city health department, returned from her initial home visit angry and upset. "Mrs. Clark's house is filthy. It's disgusting. You can't expect me to go back."

"The family's not ready for discharge," I said. "Even though the baby's six months old, he's only been on the apnea monitor for two days. There's more teaching to do."

Kathy set her nursing bag on the table. "Mrs. Clark waddles around wearing a faded t-shirt with stains on the front. She needs to lose weight. The kitchen table is covered with dirty dishes and old crayon and finger-painted drawings. Black soot's on the windowsills, and the bathroom sink has a ring around the inside. A black and white cat sleeps on the sofa."

"Anything positive?" I asked.

"The three kids are adorable. She's their mother. It's her job to keep things neat. Besides, she's been certified in CPR and used to work as an aide in a nursing home; you'd think she'd know better."

"Get yourself a cup of coffee and sit down so we can talk," I said.

***

As I waited for her, my mind flickered back to my early days as a community health nurse and my feelings of distaste when I encountered a family with a 'dirty house.' Only this person, Mrs. Gordon, was middle-aged and the primary caregiver for her husband who was wheelchair bound from a massive CVA. He slept in a hospital bed in the living room. Two small friendly but slobbering beagles often met me at the door. Because their dog hairs covered the upholstered furniture, I had to sit on a hard wooden chair in the kitchen. I felt grateful the referral was only for a monthly and as needed visit to change his Foley catheter. Another nurse had followed the family for six weeks after Mr. Gordon's discharge from a rehabilitation center. She had completed the care plan's short term goals.

Mrs. Gordon's recliner, placed next to her husband's hospital bed, had coffee stains on the armrests and seat cushion. Stray pieces of a jigsaw puzzle sat on a card table in front of the chair. Piles of romance novels rested on the floor stacked against the wall. Dirty dishes often filled the sink.

On my first two visits, I focused on Mr. Gordon and completed the physical assessment and catheter change as quickly as possible. Mrs. Gordon seldom initiated conversation and answered my questions in a perfunctory manner. Her aloof manner didn't encourage me to ask her about herself or her needs.

At a team meeting, I described my interaction with Mrs. Gordon to my teammates. Marianne, a seasoned community health nurse, said, "You were probably brought up in a neat and organized home."

I nodded, feeling embarrassed about talking about my childhood, but then relaxed when she changed the subject back to nursing. "Community health brings out our personal prejudices and stereotypes. When our minds are caught up defending our belief systems, we can withdraw emotionally and not see our patients and families clearly."

"So different from hospital nursing," I said. "I rarely got to know my patients this well."

Marianne continued. "Anytime you're critical or make a personal judgment about someone because of their lifestyle or living situation, look within yourself first. Think back to how, when, and what you learned from those around you. As children, we pick up negative stereotypes easily and quickly—ideas about religion, politics, sexual orientation, even housekeeping. Deeply engrained personal values that stereotype can interfere with care *without our awareness. We can't develop an effective care plan until we can see the problems from the patients' perspectives."*

Marianne's few simple comments changed my focus. She was right that my organized family home and my parent's belief that a dirty house equated with laziness and disrespect had compromised my care to the Gordon's. While my style of living was different than theirs, it was not necessarily better. I had subconsciously judged Mrs. Gordon as sloppy and uncaring without knowing her as a person. Only if her housekeeping negatively impacted the family's health or if Mrs. Gordon saw it as a problem, should it impact my nursing care.

On my next home visit, Mrs. Gordon agreed to sit at the kitchen table and talk. She wore a man's t-shirt and stained khaki slacks. Her shoulder length salt and pepper gray hair was pulled back into a pony tail. "You look tired today," I said.

She shrugged. "No more than usual. We're doin' okay." Her eyes filled with tears. "At least I was. I was doin' great after the other nurse left. She taught me a lot. I guess the eleven months of taking care of him have taken its toll." She pointed to the living room.

I swallowed hard realizing Mrs. Gordon wasn't lazy or disrespectful. Now I saw the person behind the aloof façade, a woman tired, anxious, and depressed. All of a sudden I understood the emotional and physical impact of being tied to the house day after day. Once I took off my smoke tinged glasses, I could see the problem clearly.

I obtained home health aide help for bathing and made a referral to the social worker for long-term planning. At my suggestion, Mrs. Gordon shared her overwhelming feelings with her two adult children and her primary physician, who prescribed an antidepressant. Mrs. Gordon refused a referral to hospice believing that there was still hope for her husband's recovery.

Housekeeping issues were never discussed; but, on subsequent visits, no dirty dishes sat in the sink and Mrs. Gordon began meeting me at the door dressed in clean clothes and with a smile on her face. "I'm back to my bowling on Wednesday mornings when the aide's here. I asked my son to help with the grocery shopping and pick up Harry's prescriptions." She shook her head. "He surprised me by agreeing to help so readily."

"You look like a different person," I said. "I'm glad you made those changes."

She nodded. "I can see Harry has slipped, ever so slightly over time. I'm thinking about having him evaluated for hospice." Tears filled her eyes.

I squeezed her hand. "Hospice nurses can keep patients like Harry comfortable. Hospice will help you, too, and your children. You have my card. Call me with any questions."

That day, I left the Gordon's home with a lighter heart, feeling grateful I had taken off my smoke tinged glasses. Now, maybe I could help Kathy take off hers.

***

Kathy had a sullen look on her face when she came back to the room and sat down. Her right foot tapped up and down under the table.

I leaned back in my chair. "There are lots of reasons for 'dirty houses'—depression, difficulty moving around, poor eyesight. Some people aren't interested in housekeeping; they like to do different things with their time."

Kathy took a pen from her pocket and rolled it between her hands. "There are twenty-four hours in a day. People need to use them wisely."

"Let me tell you about a similar situation," I said.

She listened attentively as I recounted my experience with the Gordon's. The longer I talked the more still her foot became.

"Hmm." she said after I had finished. "I do remember sitting at the dinner table listening to my dad make fun of our neighbor who was very overweight. She used to garden in shorts and an old t-shirt. Even my mom laughed at his sarcastic comments. A fat man who worked at my uncle's hardware store was really lazy."

"We pick up many of our attitudes from our childhoods. After a while we don't question why we think like we do. Do you see any similarities between Mrs. Clark and Mrs. Gordon?"

Kathy rubbed her eyes. "Even though she has a husband who helps her, Mrs. Clark is probably anxious and depressed, too. The three kids, the baby's monitor, being tied down every day. I see your point. On my next visit, I'll try to do what you did, talk to Mrs. Clark one to one."

I smiled at her. "You're not seeing through smoke tinged glasses anymore."

TWO NURSES: ONE OLD AND THE OTHER NEW

Caring is the essence if nursing.
Jean Watson

The ringing telephone jolted me awake.

"This is Dr. Watts from Shadyside Hospital calling about your mother. Yesterday, an MRI picked up a growth, about the size of a small orange, in her brain's occipital lobe. She tells me you're a nurse, so you know the protocols. I'm admitting her to the hospital immediately."

My heart did a summersault and my stomach flip-flopped. My shaky hands could barely hold a pencil steady enough to write.

Mom, a brain tumor. It couldn't be. Mom a retired nurse, a darn good one her coworkers had told me. Mom, 400 miles away.

Late the next afternoon, I arrived at the hospital to find her alone in a small semi-private room, lying in bed silently weeping. By the time our hug ended, her tears had stopped.

"Have you heard what's wrong?" she asked.

"No," I lied.

Even with my nursing background, I couldn't bear to say the words, *brain tumor.*

She fingered the bed sheets. "The doctor says I have a brain tumor. He wants to operate."

Tears filled my eyes. I squeezed her hand.

She sighed. "What happens will happen regardless of what we do."

I nodded, only partially agreeing. Old memories flashed through my mind like the moving patterns in a child's kaleidoscope. I remembered how Mom cared for Grandma when she had a stroke. Her right side had been paralyzed, and she couldn't talk or swallow normally.

Now Mom was in the hospital, unable to shower without assistance. The next morning I carried a basin of water from the bathroom to the bedside to help her wash. As I wrapped the washcloth around my fingers, I remembered my four-year-old hands splashing in a white enamel dishpan. I was helping Mom bathe my little brother. I didn't realize at the time that he was very ill. Mom squeezed red liquid medicine into his mouth from an eyedropper and then carefully peeled tape from his skin; she pulled so slowly, he didn't even flinch. When I brushed my hand across her arm, she looked at me and smiled.

Today she looked at me and smiled too.

Mom spent the next several days undergoing an extensive diagnostic work-up.

When she became restless, I tried to divert her attention. We talked about nursing and the many changes it's undergone over the years.

I smoothed out the wrinkles in her bedspread. "Remember the day I left for nursing school and asked you if you were glad to have been a nurse?"

"Of course I remember. My answer today is the same as then. Everyday I'm glad. Nursing's helped me understand what's important in life."

I nodded.

She chuckled. "You'll see. By the time you retire, if you're like me, you'll feel as if you gained more from nursing than you gave."

I fluffed her pillow. "You were right that nursing teaches you about life. It's sure helped me be a better person."

Dr. Watts explained there was a fifty-fifty chance the tumor would be cancerous with some likelihood of cardiovascular complications. I felt the blood drain from my face.

Mom seemed nonplussed. "I've stopped worrying. I'll do what I have to do."

The operation was scheduled for the next day.

While eating a late dinner in the hospital cafeteria, I saw Dr. Watts. I wanted to tell him to get a good night's rest. Instead, I nodded hello

When I walked back into Mom's room to say goodnight, she appeared to be calm sitting in a blue upholstered chair beside her bed. "Don't worry, she said. " The surgery will turn out fine, you'll see"

"I know, Mom," I lied again. "See you in the morning. Love you."

When the alarm clock awakened me the next morning, my anxiety had dissipated. Maybe the operation would be successful after all.

I arrived back at the hospital to find Mom lying on a hospital cart in the hallway, looking small and frail, so different from yesterday. She raised her head and smiled.

I kissed her cheek. "I woke up with a good feeling about the surgery."

She swallowed hard. "Me, too."

We hugged each other tightly, each of us knowing it was a moment neither of us would forget. The attendant came to wheel her into surgery. The head nurse walked with me to the surgical waiting area.

Hours later, the volunteer called me to the desk. "Your mom's out of surgery now. Dr. Watts will be down to talk to you soon." I felt my heartbeat quicken.

Fifteen minutes later, Dr. Watts burst through the door wearing wrinkled green scrubs. "We got the whole thing out. It was benign. I don't anticipate any problems. She's in the recovery room now. You can see her shortly."

Hours later I was sitting beside Mom's bed.

Her eyes fluttered opened. "You're still here?" she murmured, her head swathed in a turban of white bandages.

I squeezed her hand. "Of course. It's what you would have done."

"Two nurses, one old and the other new.

LOOKING BEYOND THE OBVIOUS

The most practical lesson that can be given to nurses is to teach them what to observe.

Florence Nightingale

Amy, the nursing supervisor at the health department, stopped by my cubicle and handed me a new referral. "He's a healthy six year old boy with Down Syndrome. No cardiac problems, but over the past two years, he's gained so much weight his body mass index is at the 90th percentile."

I pushed my charting to the side of my desk. "Is the mom overweight, too?"

"Somewhat. An older mom. She's broken two appointments this month. Can you make a home visit? Here's the physical assessment from the nurse practitioner."

***

Two days later I knocked on the family's apartment door. A stocky middle-aged woman wearing khaki slacks and a smudged white t-shirt invited me into the living room. "You must be the nurse. Amy told me you'd be coming."

After I introduced myself, she said, "I'm Linda Harris, Eric's mother. Call me Linda." She ran her fingers through her short brown hair gray at the temples.

"And this must be Eric?" I waved in his direction. Dressed in a navy sweat suit, Eric sat in the corner of the room in an oversized children's rocking chair watching *Sesame Street* on television.

Piles of men and women's clothes were stacked on the sofa near a sewing machine by the back wall. "I'm a seamstress," she said when she saw me looking at the clothing.

"You're busy then," I said.

"People bring me their clothes. They want this, and then they want that. I, uh, I have to work. We need the extra money."

After washing my hands in their small bathroom, I sat down on the sofa beside the clothes piles. "Let's talk a bit."

"Amy convinced me to let you come, but there's nothin' a nurse can help with. Eric's my baby. He's doin' okay, so what if he has a little baby fat."

"He's really not a baby anymore," I said.

Linda swallowed hard. "You don't know what it's like. I'm here every afternoon with him. Some mornings, too, when he doesn't go to school."

"I can imagine."

She sighed. "Eric's a sweetie. He sits here with me watching television while I sew. He loves to sit and eat. I know it's bad for him but…" Tears filled her eyes as she walked over and put her hands on his shoulders.

Eric's soft straight brown hair had a crooked part on one side. A box of *Cheezits* sat on the table beside him. I walked over to his chair. He smiled at me behind his wire-rimmed glasses. "Want a cookie?" he asked holding an outstretched palm with four *Cheezits*.

"Thank you, but I'm not hungry now." Spotting several blocks in the corner of the room, I asked, "Do you want to build a tower?"

He readily agreed and giggled when our stack of four blocks fell over.

Linda laughed.

I smiled at her. "Most mothers want to feed their children well. Eating can be an emotional thing, too. But often, more isn't better."

I learned Linda and her husband, Stan, felt overwhelmed with the care responsibilities of their son even though they had adjusted to the fact that he would never be a normal child. He worked long hours as a security guard and while a gentle man, he kept emotionally detached from the family and was never present during my visits. Linda believed Eric was happy but admitted his extra weight could compromise his health.

The child was a cheerful affectionate boy, short and heavy for his age, and prone to upper respiratory infections. Although toilet trained, he had poor muscle tone and a lumbering gait. His tongue protruded slightly. No physical problems were evident. Developmentally, he functioned as a three year old.

***

On the next home visit, I said, "Baby fat isn't always good. Obese children tend to have weight problems all their lives. Childhood habits are hard to break."

Linda smoothed her t-shirt over her stomach. "Maybe I don't watch what he eats well enough. I love him though. It was hard at first finding out he was different, but he's so sweet and loving. What else can I do?"

"Let's write down some ideas."

Linda got up to get a pencil and paper.

"You go first, something you think could help," I said.

"Maybe not giving him the *Snickers* bar after supper."

"We'll write that down as number one," I said.

Together, we developed the rest of the care plan. She agreed to complete a three-day food diary for Eric, including his snacks. From the diary I determined the family's food preferences and coordinated my suggestions with their eating style. According to the Food Pyramid, the family's regular meals contained too many servings of breads and milk and not enough servings of fruits and vegetables. Although his protein intake was adequate, Eric's snacks, *Snickers* bars, *Cheezits*, *Oreo* cookies, and chocolate milk shakes, pushed his caloric intake over the 1,800 per day recommendation.

The overall goals were for Eric to maintain his present weight until it was within the normal range for his age and to eat foods daily from each of the major food groups.

Linda agreed to a referral to a Food Stamp program, which allowed her to purchase more fresh fruits and vegetables. Using nutritional handouts, I taught her healthier food choices and gave her pamphlets with *Heart Healthy* recipes. She prepared more low calorie, low fat meals that included fruits, vegetables, and whole grains.

To encourage Eric's independence and physical activity, Linda enrolled him in an afternoon playgroup for developmentally delayed children and spent time with him every day in a one-on-one activity. On Saturdays, Stan, Linda, and Eric went grocery shopping. The parents compared food labels and let Eric participate in choosing healthy foods. Sunday afternoons the three of them often went to a nearby park.

Linda declined referrals to a nutritionist and the local chapter of the National Association for Down Syndrome but agreed to keep the phone numbers handy for future reference.

**

On my last visit, a smiling Eric met me at the door with a block in each hand. Linda had limited his television watching to two hours a day and replaced his candy and cookie snacks with a granola bar or a small dish of dry cereal, yogurt, or raisins. She'd started making his milk shakes at home with a blender using skim milk and fruit juice instead of buying them at a fast food restaurant.

Before I said good-bye, an excited Linda exclaimed, "Stan and I are losing weight and have more energy. We feel more like a family now."

**

Working with the Harris' made me realize the complexity of family health problems. Nurses must stay flexible and creative and look beyond the obvious to find long-term solutions. Including referrals to community resources in the care plan broadens the base of support for the family and increases the likelihood the mutually set goals will be met and maintained.

KEEPING HOPE ALIVE

Live life when you have it. Life is a splendid gift—there is nothing small about it.

Florence Nightingale

It was my first nursing visit to Thad and Larissa Meyers. The three of us sat around their kitchen table discussing how to best manage an exacerbation of Thad's multiple sclerosis. Tears welled in the corners of Larissa's brown eyes, as she twisted a strand of her strawberry blonde hair around her finger.

"His MS seemed to get worse overnight," Larissa said. He can't walk up the stairs anymore without hanging onto the railing for dear life. Dr. Downing says it's time for a stair lift."

"I can beat these new problems," Thad replied. "Prayer, persistence, and exercise. My sales manager at Acme Foods suggested a disability leave, but I refused. Give me a month here at home. I'll show him." His hands shook as he hitched his belt over his potbelly. "There will be no damn chair lift in my house. Mind over matter."

Larissa sighed. "He needs to retire, stay home and rest, and let me take care of him. I've lost twenty pounds in the last three months worrying about him."

I took a deep breath, remembering that the physician referral documented an exacerbation of an aggressive form of MS that limited the chance of significant recovery. Double vision accentuated his mobility problems.

Hope and unrealistic expectations, a common but difficult scenario I'd often seen in my work as a home health care nurse.

But how to help Thad accept his limitations but keep hope in his heart. And convince Larissa to encourage her husband to be as independent as possible. Larissa, like many caregivers, enabled her husband, making him feel useless. The barriers to realistic goal setting ran through my mind—denial, anger, fear, lack of knowledge, and lack of social supports. First I needed to do a complete assessment and work with the couple to develop an effective long-term care plan with an overall goal and the individual steps to accomplish it. Without realistic expectations, Thad and Larissa's fears and anger would further the family dysfunction.

I paused. "Thad, physical therapy can strengthen your muscles and improve your walking. An occupational therapist can teach you ways to deal with the small things like brushing your teeth and shaving."

"I've already had two stints with them and learned everything I need to know. Could teach them a thing or two." He clenched his fists.

"But the stair lift. I want a stair lift installed now. Otherwise, he'll fall," Larissa said in a trembling voice.

I looked at Thad. "Let's make a deal. You agree to have physical and occupational therapy for four weeks and I'll visit twice a week, communicate with the doctor, and follow up on any problems you have. Then, we'll talk about the stair lift."

"God, another session! I wanted to do it myself this time." He ran his hand over his forehead. "Oh, all right."

***

Over the next month, I counseled Thad and Larissa, individually and as a couple.

"I'm scared what will happen to me if Thad dies," Larissa admitted one day while we were alone reviewing several handouts on managing the disease.

"That's understandable but overprotecting him and not letting him do what he can safely hurts his rehab potential." I highlighted sections in the pamphlets that pertained to caregiving.

She frowned. "I'm angry at him for getting sick and feel guilty about that, too. We're only fifty-five. If he got hurt, I'd blame myself. That's why I'm overprotective. I'm scared."

I nodded. "All your feelings are normal. Most caregivers feel the same."

"No one else I know has to deal with MS. I'm alone, depressed."

"The Multiple Sclerosis Society has a caregiver support group that meets every week at the city library. That's where you'll find people who feel just like you. Talking with them will help."

***

Thad expectations for the future also were unrealistic. His fear and anger manifested in denial instead of depression.

"My vision has improved with the new medication. My legs are stronger after finishing my stint with PT. I tried to go upstairs without my walker yesterday, almost made it. Then, I slipped on the steps, scraped my knee. Damn steps. Now Larissa's really bugging me about the chair lift."

"It's hard to get the mind and the body working together sometimes. With a chair lift, you could save your energy for things that are important and that you enjoy."

"Like going to work?"

"That could be a realistic goal. What about cutting back to three days a week?"

He smiled. "I can live with that. And Larissa's right. The stair lift is a good idea."

***

Helping clients set realistic goals is important to keep hope alive. Unrealistic goals foster fear, denial, anger, and depression.

Without hope, clients lose the moorings for their lives.

NURSES KNOW

The trained nurse has become one of the great blessings of humanity taking a place beside the physician and the priest.

William Osler, MD

Over the years, nurses' responsibilities have changed dramatically, but their important role in maintaining quality patient care has remained constant. Nurses were there for me in 1976 after I was injured in a serious automobile accident.

***

Somewhere in the distance an ambulance siren shrieked. Was I dreaming? No. But where was I? Sensing something was seriously wrong, I shook my head and opened my eyes. Why was I lying in a field of long grass and weeds? When the fog lifted, I remembered that I'd been driving home from the Visiting Nurse Association on a lazy country road. There was a crash and my world went dead.

A thin middle-aged woman with straggly gray hair stood over me. The shocked look in her dark brown eyes that conveyed fear, pity, and horror surprised me. I sat up and methodically flexed my legs, toes, fingers, and arms, feeling thankful that they moved. My right thumb tingled; it was hard to move my left arm, but it didn't hurt or tingle. I'd broken my left clavicle, I thought.

I smelled smoke. "How did I get here?"

She pointed to a man standing beside her. "We pulled you from the car, afraid the engine would explode."

Minutes later a policeman arrived. "The cement truck coming the other way lost control; he got you broadside,"

An EMT lifted me onto a stretcher and transported me to a nearby hospital's emergency room. Unreality persisted; it wasn't really me who'd been injured. A nurse, Sheila, helped move me to a gurney. Dr. Philips, a calm middle-aged doctor, examined me and talked in a gentle reassuring manner. I appreciated his compassion.

He fingered the pen in his lab coat pocket. "Nothing is seriously wrong, just some scrapes and bruises. I'm going to order a complete set of body x-rays."

Twenty minutes later I was transferred to the X-Ray Department. I was X-rayed lying down, sitting on a round stool, and standing. I was thankful to be able to stand but wondered if I should be on my feet.

Just as I was asked to get up for the second time, Sheila's voice resonated from the hallway. "She could have a spinal injury. Don't move her from the gurney!"

Thank God, somebody has some brains, I thought. Mine sure weren't working. The X-ray technicians quickly transferred me back to the padded hospital cart. *Nurses know basic first aid guidelines.*

After I was returned to the emergency room, Dr. Philips reappeared. "Have you ever had a neck injury?" he asked.

"No, never." My heart flip-flopped.

He took a deep breath. "The X-rays show a slight fracture of a cervical vertebra. It can be easily treated."

"Tell me more. I'm a nurse."

"The fracture is at C-6 with a slight anterior subluxation. A week or ten days in traction and then a neck brace for a couple of months should do it."

His words comforted me. Sheila placed a stiff collar on my neck and sandbags on each side of my head.

I was transferred to the neurological unit, where a resident met me. "I'm going to drill little holes in each side of your head right above your ear to set up the traction."

I gasped. "How many times have you done this before?"

He didn't answer but focused on his surgical set up.

My stomach churned. "Let me think." I looked at Joanne, the nurse assisting him.

She understood my concern. "Mike, let's page the Senior Resident."

He nodded. The senior resident came and assisted Mike insert the tongs. I cringed at the sound of the drill boring through my skull. When the weights were attached to the tongs, tears filled my eyes.

Joanne held my hand through the fifteen-minute ordeal. "We're here for you. Try to relax. You're doing very well." *Nurses know how to act as client advocates and reassure patients.*

The next day I was examined by a neurosurgeon, Dr. Malik. He looked directly at me. "I suggest surgery to fuse your C-6 vertebrae using a hip bone graft, then putting you in a Minerva Jacket upper body cast for six weeks."

I felt the blood drain from my face. "That's the only option?"

"That's the best option. We'll need to keep you in traction and wait a week for the swelling to subside."

My mind tumbled with anxiety—infection, permanent paralysis, a blood clot, but, after talking with my family, I agreed. I wanted the surgery to be over quickly. Completely bedridden I could only lie on my back. Nurses' aides bathed, repositioned me every few hours, and fed me. My shoulder length hair was braided into five plaits.

The morning of the surgery, a technician came to my room to transport me to the operating room. As she started to remove the weights from my head, I said, "The weights have to stay on. They keep my spine straight."

My husband concurred and called the nurse, Paige. She insisted the weights stay in place for the transfer, and the technician complied. *Nurses know how to keep patients safe.*

After the surgery I again had to lie flat in bed for another week to allow for the surgical swelling to resolve. I was bored and discouraged. Beside my family, friend, and co-worker visitors, I was reassured by the nurse's chit-chat. They even broke the rules and allowed my young children to visit. *Nurses know how to provide emotional support.*

A favorite nurse was Karen. "Another few days and you'll have your body cast. Then you'll be able to get up and walk."

I scratched my neck. "Hallelujah. I never thought this day would come."

Finally my stitches were removed and plans were made for the Minerva Jacket application. I was taken to the cast room for the procedure and then returned to my bed. At first the absence of the traction and the damp warm plaster on my chest, back of my head and neck, and around my forehead comforted me. As time passed and the plaster cooled, I began to shiver with a bone-chilling cold no blanket could ease. Even though the cast extended to my pelvis, now I could sit up using the handset on my electric hospital bed.

I ran my fingers over an oily braid that stuck out of the six-inch circular open area on my scalp's crown; my hair hadn't been shampooed for two weeks. When Karen came into my room later, she said, "You can go home tomorrow."

"I can't wait."

Karen nodded. "Would you like a shampoo before you're discharged?"

I smiled. "I'd love that."

She rolled a hospital cart into the room, and I squiggled onto it. She wheeled me into the utility room, covered my cast with a plastic bag, loosened the braids, and washed my hair. Then she re-braided it into a single plait protruding from a round opening in my cast on the top of my head.

"That feels wonderful." I said. *Nurses know the importance of personal comfort.*

***

My competent nurses practiced in 1976. Today's nurses work in a much more intense high-tech environment and follow evidenced-based practice guidelines, but they continue to be client advocates and act to keep patients comfortable and safe. They remain the backbone of our country's health care system.

WHAT NURSING TAUGHT US

Education is the most powerful weapon which you can use to change the world.

Nelson Mandela

"Plan a trip to LA?" Cindy, my old friend from nursing school, wrote in an e-mail. It had been years since I'd seen her. Months later I was flying across the country for a visit.

Even though we had been in different specialties, she in psychiatric nursing and I in community health, the bond we shared as young student nurses stayed strong through the years. Since our graduation, we never lived in the same city, yet our lives crisscrossed many times through the years—weddings, funerals, and long vacation week-ends. We learned about important life changes through scribbled letters and erratic phone calls. Thanks to what nursing taught us about people, we knew the challenges the other was experiencing. The empathy between us never died; we heard the music behind each other's remarks.

***

She met me outside the secure area of the airport. A broad smile lit up her face. "Lo, It's so good to see you."

I stood back to look at her. The way she styled her short brown hair hadn't changed. The skin around her eyes was a little softer, and like me, she was a few pounds heavier, but she hadn't lost her sense of style. Trendy jeans, a black silk blouse, loop earrings, and *Teva* sandals so different from the student nurses' shoes and navy blue uniforms with white aprons we wore so long ago. Had it not been for nursing school, I never would have met her. We were reared in different states in families with vastly different value systems. *Nursing is what held us together.*

As she welcomed me into her home, memories of our three years together in nursing school tumbled through my head like a twirling child's kaleidoscope. Anatomy class when we looked through a microscope to watch the cells in the blood of a frog's artery spurt along with the beat of his heart. Nursing arts labs where we practiced our newly learned skills on manikins. Clinical rotations under the ever watchful eyes of our instructors, reciting pertinent facts about medications that we were to have memorized from our drug cards, keeping our hands from shaking as we learned to give our first IM injections, and computing the correct amount of medication to add to a patient's IV. Struggling over term papers and sharing notes from our three-hour Monday and Wednesday lectures. *Nursing was instrumental in developing our critical thinking skills.*

Soon, we were sitting at her dining room table sipping tea. She leaned forward. "Back then, did you ever think we'd still be meeting like this today?"

I picked up my cup. "It never entered my mind. On our first day of school, you stood next to me in the dorm lobby waiting for an elevator. We talked briefly. Your smile made me relax. I was shy and scared."

She wrapped her tea bag round her spoon. "I was scared, too, but didn't show it. We were so young and so different. You were quiet, smiled a lot, and blended into the woodwork. I had something to say about everything and didn't care who heard it. Somehow, I knew we would become friends."

"Yeah, we were always there to support each other, the person behind the other's back." *Nursing took our caring tendencies and made them strong. It taught us the definition of commitment.*

I rubbed my forehead. "All the things we thought important back then—having a boyfriend, outwitting the housemother, staying out after curfew. Remember our girlhood dreams of everlasting love of husbands and children. Who would have thought our lives would have taken the turns they did?"

She sighed. "We had no clue what was involved in making relationships work. We just knew we were going to live happily ever after." *Nursing taught us how our present behavior is affected by our past experiences.*

We listened intently as we rehashed the details of our early lives, intuitively sensing both the sadness each of us felt about our broken dreams and the gratefulness that we were given second chances to make things right. *Nursing taught us therapeutic communication skills; our patients helped us integrate them into our personalities and learn to trust our intuitions.*

"Remember how we crammed over the library's medical books to find the causes, treatment, and management of the different diseases?" she said. *Nursing taught us the importance of using scientific research and a comprehensive knowledge base to solve problems.*

I nodded. "And how we talked about a Higher Power and the meaning of life. We were such searchers." *Nursing taught us to look for meaning in everyday life and explore the cause-effect relationships of health and disease. Our patients taught us what really is important in life—health, family, friends, meaningful work.*

"Nursing put food on my kid's table," she added.

"Nursing kept me strong, gave me a focus," I said. "I can't imagine my life without it."

She agreed. "You know, our lives took a similar professional track without us planning it." *Nursing taught us how to set goals. It gave us the springboard to create satisfying and productive careers.*

***

Our time together passed quickly. As I sat in the airport waiting to board my plane back home, I realized how much wisdom we'd gained from each other, our patients, and our co-workers. *Nursing provided the strong bond that held our friendship together, and it gave us a secure base on which to build a meaningful personal and professional life.*

AUTHOR INFORMATION

Lois Gerber, RN, BSN, MPH believes in the spirit of community health nursing—it focus on wellness, relationships, families, and communities. Her Bachelor of Nursing degree from the University of Pittsburgh and her Master in Public Health degree and Specialist in Aging certificate from the University of Michigan opened many professional doors. In 1993, she received the Excellence in Nursing Practice Award by the Kappa Iota chapter of Sigma Theta Tau, an international nursing honor society.

As a child, Lois loved to read and write and was especially inspired by Helen Wells' Cherry Ames book series on nurses practicing in the various nursing specialties. Pearl Buck and her focus on culture and family dynamics was another of her favorite authors.

In Ohio and Michigan, Lois worked as a staff nurse and care coordinator in home health agencies, public health departments, and an Area Agency on Aging. She taught nursing students at the university level for twenty four years. For eleven years, through her geriatric care management service, she counseled families dealing with elder care issues, developed care plans for their frail members, and monitored their living situations. Her goal was to provide individualized care and keep the patient safe and as independent as possible.

For forty some years, Lois has served people of all ages, various religions and ethnicities, and different socio-economic levels. These stories reflect her experiences.